# PAVE YOUR WAY WITH CHRONIC ILLNESS

*from the same author*

**How to Do Life with a Chronic Illness**
Reclaim Your Identity, Create Independence, and Find Your Way Forward
*Pippa Stacey*
ISBN 978 1 80501 017 3
eISBN 978 1 80501 018 0
AUDIOBOOK ISBN 978 1 39981 633 5

*of related interest*

**All Tangled Up in Autism and Chronic Illness**
A Guide to Navigating Multiple Conditions
*Charli Clement*
ISBN 978 1 83997 524 0
eISBN 978 1 83997 525 7
AUDIOBOOK ISBN 978 1 39982 111 7

**Go Your Crohn Way**
A Gutsy Guide to Living with Crohn's Disease
*Kathleen Nicholls*
ISBN 978 1 84819 316 1
eISBN 978 0 85701 268 5

# PAVE YOUR WAY WITH CHRONIC ILLNESS

A Self-Discovery Journal

**Pippa Stacey**

*Illustrated by Victoria Barron*

Jessica Kingsley Publishers
London and Philadelphia

First published in Great Britain in 2025 by Jessica Kingsley Publishers
An imprint of John Murray Press

1



A CIP catalogue record for this title is available from the British Library and the Library of Congress

ISBN 978 1 80501 749 3
eISBN 978 1 80501 750 9

Printed and bound in Great Britain by Bell & Bain Limited

Jessica Kingsley Publishers' policy is to use papers that are natural, renewable and recyclable products and made from wood grown in sustainable forests. The logging and manufacturing processes are expected to conform to the environmental regulations of the country of origin.

Jessica Kingsley Publishers
Carmelite House
50 Victoria Embankment
London EC4Y 0DZ

www.jkp.com

John Murray Press
Part of Hodder & Stoughton Ltd
An Hachette Company

The authorised representative in the EEA is Hachette Ireland,
8 Castlecourt Centre, Dublin 15, D15 XTP3, Ireland (email: info@hbgi.ie)

# CONTENTS

# A NOTE FROM THE AUTHOR

As we all know, chronic illness is unique. No two people are impacted in the same way, and the differences in lifestyle between those more 'mildly' affected and those more severely affected can be stratospheres away from each other.

I've endeavoured to be as mindful as possible about this spectrum while creating this journal, but it's likely you will come across sections or activities that feel more relevant to you than others. My condition affects me every single day and has done for the last decade, but I have never been housebound or bedbound for prolonged periods the way that others in the chronic illness community have. Therefore, I've tried to share ways of thinking and adapting that hold widespread value, while making sure I'm not speaking for those whose lived experiences are very different from my own.

No matter who you are or what has led you here, I hope you will find meaning and comfort throughout this journal. There may be parts that feel as if they were written for you, but others that you vehemently disagree with. And that's okay – there is no one-size-fits-all approach when it comes to chronic illness. I encourage you to take in the advice that you find helpful, and let the other stuff gently pass you by. That stuff may be what somebody else in different circumstances needs instead.

I'm truly honoured that you've picked up this journal, and that you're using your valuable energy to read it. The content of these pages is not a substitute for medical advice or care, but I hope it holds plenty of positive benefits for your broader lifestyle and reminds you (yes, you!) of the brilliant person you are. Let's do this!

# FOREWORD

Since Pippa Stacey's first book, *University and Chronic Illness: A Survival Guide* (2020), I have been captivated by her way of writing which speaks to a chronically ill audience. Her work reminds us that lived experience is paramount when connecting to readers. I had the pleasure of being a contributor to her second book, *How to Do Life with a Chronic Illness* (2024). Again, this book spoke to her audience in a way that is captivating, moving and informative. Pippa's new book, *Pave Your Way with Chronic Illness*, is no different.

As a therapist who is chronically ill working with chronically ill individuals, I am constantly seeking new ways to enhance the quality of life for both myself and my clients in an accessible way. This book has significantly aided my personal journey with chronic illness and has led to important shifts in my counselling practice. I have incorporated the activities outlined in Pippa's book into my therapy sessions and eagerly anticipate recommending it to clients as a valuable workbook to complement their therapeutic experiences.

One of the standout features of this book is its accessibility. Pippa demonstrates a nuanced understanding of diverse needs, allowing readers to approach the material in a way that suits them best. For example, she categorises activities into 'low,' 'medium,' and 'better' battery questions, enabling readers to select tasks that align with their energy levels at any given time. As someone who is autistic, I also find the book to be neurodiversity-affirming and accommodating for those who are COVID-conscious.

From my training as a therapist, I subscribe to the idea that checking in with oneself regularly is extremely helpful in monitoring emotional responses and can help ground a person. This concept is woven throughout the book, particularly in the 'time capsule' activity, where readers can record their thoughts and feelings regarding their health and any emotions that come up while engaging with the content.

A particular aspect of this book I enjoyed was how it encourages the reader to reconnect with their personal identity. I understand that having a chronic illness can make me feel disconnected from who I am as a person. Countless doctor appointments have, at times, made me feel medicalised. This book powerfully reminds me that it's okay to explore all aspects of my identity, helping me to revive and embrace them.

My favourite section of this book was *Section 4 – Create Your Happy Place*. This section helps the reader discover 'what makes their heart happy' and then uses activities and journal prompts to help the reader implement these elements into their lives while practising pacing. I also like how there is an activity to encourage the reader to make their space feel more like '*you*' in an inclusive way while acknowledging the limitations people may face.

Something I have noticed is that my chronically ill clients struggle with thinking about the future. This usually is because it can feel too overwhelming to imagine any kind of positive future when their chronic illness causes them suffering. *Section 6 – Thoughts for the Future* gently encourages the reader to imagine what they would like their future to look like within the boundaries of their circumstances. The way this section's activities are structured allows the reader to connect with the emotions they have about the future and tentatively give prompts to create ideas for goals they may have all while being chronic illness-friendly. One of the final activities in this book is to 'write a letter to your future self.' This exercise fosters self-reflection and instils a sense of connection to the idea of a future, emphasising hope and personal growth.

In conclusion, Pippa Stacey's *Pave Your Way with Chronic Illness* is a vital resource that resonates deeply with individuals with chronic illness. Through its accessible and engaging format, the book not only provides journal prompts and activities that encourage self-reflection and personal growth but also fosters a sense of community among readers by providing resources for building connections with others. By weaving personal narratives, validating emotional experiences, and promoting the exploration of identity, it empowers individuals to reclaim their sense of self and envision a hopeful future. This book is more than just a workbook; it's a companion on the journey of living with chronic illness, reminding us that we are not alone and that there is room for joy, connection, and hope in our lives. For anyone seeking to enhance their quality of life while navigating chronic illness, *Pave Your Way with Chronic Illness* is an invaluable book worth reading.

*Charlotte Elizabeth Beaumont*

Registered Member: 387024
British Association for Counselling and Psychotherapy
charlotteelizabethcounselling.com
Instagram: @counsellingwithchar
charlotteelizabethcounselling@gmail.com

# INTRODUCTION

WELCOME to *Pave Your Way with Chronic Illness*!

This journal is designed to be a safe and inviting space for people living with chronic illnesses and/or long-term health conditions. Throughout these pages, you'll find creative prompts, engaging activities, time capsules for self-reflection, spaces for thought-dumping, and so much more. Each section is designed to help you reconnect with yourself, identify the things that bring you joy, and consider how you can take steps towards leading a life that truly feels like your own again.

In my previous book, *How to Do Life with a Chronic Illness*, I aimed to steer the narrative away from the physical elements of long-term conditions (like symptom tracking and medication options) that often dominate the conversation. As much as I wish it were otherwise, this journal cannot and will not claim to have any impact on your level of illness or steps towards physical recovery. Instead, however, we will focus on getting to know yourself *alongside* your chronic illness. Each page will acknowledge and validate the life-altering experience you are living through, while gently inviting you to reflect on broader aspects of your identity and wellbeing too. We'll approach this by exploring your sense of self and your current lifestyle, developing your self-advocacy skills and levels of resilience, creating space for the things that bring you happiness, considering the value of positive relationships with others, making accessible intentions and future plans, and so much more. And, spoiler alert, there are colouring pages in here too. Because what situation in life can't be improved by a nice bit of colouring?

When you have a chronic illness, it can feel as though so much choice and autonomy has been taken away from you. We have to adapt our ways of existing in almost every conceivable way, and navigate all kinds of physical and societal barriers in the world around us. Often, it feels as if we have to fight so hard to be heard and access the support we require that there's barely any energy or brain space left over for ourselves. There are many things that are outside our control – our disease trajectory, the support we have access to, the systemic ableism all around us... I know that, sometimes, anything we do to try and help ourselves can feel futile; as if we're fighting a losing battle. The feelings of hopelessness that can come with that can be crushing, and the day those barriers are finally broken down and disability inclusion is achieved cannot come soon enough.

Let me be clear – this journal is not designed to minimise those experiences or promote toxic positivity. You will find no patient-blaming here, or a pushing of the outdated narrative that any challenge in life can be overcome with a positive attitude. From my own lived experiences, I know that even with all the will in the world, you cannot change your body's anatomy simply by thinking positively and squashing down the tough stuff. If that were true, it's likely that I wouldn't be here writing this, and you wouldn't be here reading this. The fact that you're living with a long-term condition is *not* a reflection on your strength of character or diligence as a human being.

That's why I want to posit an alternative approach here instead. Many of us have learned that our illness trajectories are very rarely linear. Even when you have a clear end goal in sight, there's rarely a straight or predetermined journey forward towards your destination. On the cover of my previous book, you may have noticed a winding path in the background of the text. It's there because over the last decade, I've come to accept that doing anything in life with an energy-limiting condition is rarely straightforward, and I've become much better equipped to navigate the squiggles and setbacks along the way. But although I often wish the path were a little smoother, I now know that the quirks and intricacies of it are a powerful part of what makes me unique. They have truly shaped the person I am today, and I'm willing to bet they've shaped the person you are too.

I chose the title *Pave Your Way with Chronic Illness* for this journal because I want to empower you to embrace your own squiggly path too. It's not about pushing your condition to the kerbside or pretending it doesn't exist, but taking small and sustainable steps towards a life that feels uniquely yours. Rather than seeing physical progress or recovery as the end goal, which is something we don't have a great deal of conscious control over, what about if we remove the focus from the medical management of chronic illness and think about our broader lives and identity instead?

## A bit about me

My name is Pippa, and I live in Yorkshire. For the first 15-ish years of my life, I was a very active person. I loved to dance and was in pre-professional ballet training, I enjoyed other energetic hobbies like trampolining, I was often volunteering and fundraising for charities in my free time, and I was without a doubt one of those neurotic Type A kids who's always on the go and eager to please. For the most part, I enjoyed school and got grades I was happy with, and I loved spending my free time with friends.

My early symptoms of chronic illness were subtle, setting in slowly and gradually. I visited my GP many times over the years to try and find answers and discuss actionable ways to feel better, only to be met with a good dollop of condescension and medical gaslighting. I poured so much of the energy I had left into holding on to my previous identity, resisting change with all my might. However, after a significant relapse at the age of 19, emulating my former self became completely impossible. I was diagnosed with myalgic encephalomyelitis/chronic fatigue syndrome (ME/CFS), and sent back home to my childhood bedroom to figure out the rest for myself.

For a good few years following my diagnosis, I was so consumed with the physical and mental struggle of my situation that it felt as if there wasn't much room in my life for anything else. On the surface, I was still trying to carry on like any non-disabled person, completing my university education and trying to maintain existing relationships, but internally I felt completely lost.

You can read more about my experiences of adapting to chronic illness and finding ways to chase joy in my previous book and the predecessor to this journal, *How to Do Life with a Chronic Illness*. I wrote the book to provide comfort and advice for anybody going through similar struggles, just as I've created this journal to help anybody wanting to further that journey and reconnect with their sense of identity too.

Through my lived experiences and over a decade of trial and error, I've become much more skilled at managing my disability and finding accessible ways to do the things I want to do – well, as much as is possible alongside a fluctuating condition. However, something I've always found more difficult is keeping in tune with myself and who I really am as a person. When so many of your formative young adult years have been dictated by surviving and getting through, you can end up feeling like a 'professional patient': as if your identity begins and ends with your medical diagnosis. And when you have an energy-limiting condition that restricts your ability to do the things you love and feel like your truest self, it's no surprise that you can end up feeling disorientated.

As I spoke about in my previous book, I feel that incorporating disability and/or chronic illness into your identity can be a powerful thing. Many of us are made to feel as though we need to squash down our reality or pretend it doesn't affect us as much as it does, or that being open and realistic about our conditions somehow makes us more complacent in the struggles we face. Let me tell you right now, those incorrect assumptions have no place here. This journal will recognise and affirm the very real challenges you are facing all the way through...but it will go one step further to help you explore your broader life and identity at the same time. I have been a human guinea pig for all the activities within these pages, and I hope that working your way through them will feel as comforting and enjoyable for you as it has for me.

## How to use this journal

This journal is divided into six sections. Each section contains a few pages of information and lived experiences from me, followed by a diverse range of accessible and creative activities. These activities differ in theme and format throughout each section, but are divided into three key elements: 'low battery' questions for when you're having a tougher symptom day, 'medium battery' questions for when you're around your baseline, and 'better battery' questions for when you have the time and bandwidth to really think about and consider your answers. You'll also find regular 'time capsule' pages between sections, where you can thought-dump your emotions and the things that are happening in your life as you experience them in real time.

Speaking of time, there is no set period in which you're encouraged to complete this journal, nor is there a daily obligation or routine to commit to if you want to get the most out of it. These activities are designed to be completed at a time, place, and pace that suits you. You may like to complete just one activity a day, or do a few at a time. You can go about things in whatever way feels best to you, though I would encourage you to explore the sections chronologically rather than jumping ahead.

There's plenty of room to write, doodle, and annotate in this book, or you could set aside a notebook or online document to engage with the activities if this is more accessible for you.

You can download editable PDF versions of all the interactive elements of this journal (including the 'battery' questions, 'time capsule' pages, and the letter to your future self) at **https://digitalhub.jkp.com/redeem** using the code **TELYNLM**. You can also download extra copies of the colouring pages here if you want to enjoy them again!

And remember, each activity deliberately allows for creativity and your own interpretation – there is no right or wrong way to complete anything. However, to truly get the most out of this experience, I recommend giving yourself some time and space to really indulge in the process. Make yourself your favourite hot drink, and if you can, set your phone on 'do not disturb' for a little while. This space is completely yours, and I can't wait for you to get started.

Are you ready? Let us begin...

# TIME CAPSULE 1

Use this space to record information about you, your chronic illness, and your health and wellbeing at this moment in time. You'll have the opportunity to do this throughout the book, so you can keep in tune with how your thoughts or feelings are evolving.

**What is the date and time?**

**How is your physical health today?**

**How is your mental health today?**

**What are three things you feel grateful for today?**

**What challenges are you facing at the moment?**

**Time to thought-dump. What's on your mind today?**

## SECTION 1

# LET'S TALK ABOUT YOU

SOMETIMES it can feel as though our chronic illnesses completely eclipse our personal identity. When so much of your time and resources must be allocated to managing your condition, it may feel as though there's zero energy left in the tank to explore your sense of 'you-ness'.

During the early years of my chronic illness, I internalised the idea that being a sick person or patient was my primary identity. It felt as if the only way things could be different would be if I experienced a full recovery and returned to being exactly the same person as I was before. However, as the years passed and this full recovery failed to materialise, I realised that there had to be another way. How could I start feeling like myself again, while living with something that had altered my sense of self so significantly?

Our identity is defined as the way we see ourselves and present that self to the wider world, and it's made up of a broad range of things. First of all, there's the demographic information about ourselves – our gender, sexuality, ethnicity, socio-economic status, and many other elements that can impact the way we see ourselves and how we interact with the world. However, our sense of identity is also shaped by our passions, beliefs, and values in life. Although we don't have conscious control over our demographics, such as who we love or the colour of our skin, we do have some autonomy over our likes and dislikes and the way we express ourselves.

There are huge variations in quality of life between people affected severely by chronic illness and those affected less severely, but no matter where you fall on this spectrum, the chances are that your way of life now looks very different to how it once did. You may feel as though your personality and the way that you perceive the world has been radically altered by living with your condition. You may have had to lose or reduce the activities that once shaped your identity and the way you spend your time because of your symptoms. Your values and relationships with others may have been tested and shaken, leaving you feeling lost or isolated as you try and find a way forward. These are really difficult things to go through, and let it be said right now that the pain and grief you may be feeling because of these things is completely valid.

That's why I'm of the opinion that it's completely okay for chronic illness to form part of your identity. For me, and likely for you, my condition has too much prominence over every element of my life for it to be otherwise. However, despite what the media may have told us in the past, adopting disability and/or chronic illness into your identity isn't inherently a negative thing. We're often consumed by the ways our condition might have made life harder or feel more out of our control...but believe it or not (I didn't believe it for a very long time at first!), there are many ways that chronic illness can positively influence your identity too. In my experience, living with an energy-limiting condition has strengthened my resilience, made me a more creative thinker, and given me a much deeper sense of empathy for others. Although I could have done without the disabling symptoms that came as a package deal with them, I am genuinely grateful for these qualities.

Of course, not everybody will feel the same way. You may have picked up this journal because you want to cast chronic illness to the sidelines of your life as much as humanly possible. Identity is unique, and everybody is entitled to their opinion about whether or not their health condition should have a place in it. But for me, embracing my chronic illness as part of my identity has been one of the most empowering experiences of my life.

Perhaps you have been afraid to reflect on your identity in the wake of your diagnosis. When I was at my most unwell, I was very resistant to the idea that I could still feel like myself while going through such a life-altering experience. I believed that anybody who insisted I could clearly didn't understand how debilitating my condition was or how much I had lost. Add to this the fact that many of us face stigma and gaslighting from medical professionals, and there's also the worry that trying to broaden your life or chase happiness could be weaponised against you or used as 'evidence' that your condition isn't as disabling as you say it is. The sooner we can create a society that discredits this idea, the better. I wish I'd learned sooner that joy, purpose, and a sense of self can co-exist even with a debilitating health condition. Feeling more like yourself won't rid you of your physical symptoms, but it can provide an immense sense of relief for your mental and emotional wellbeing.

Over the last decade, I've become much more comfortable and at peace with my disabled identity. This isn't something you can rush or fast-track, but I hope this section helps you to reach this point in a much timelier and more energy-efficient way than it happened for me. It's not about compelling you to go out and desperately scramble for a new identity – quite the opposite, actually. The following questions are designed to help you explore your sense of self alongside your health condition. They may lead you down some new lines of thought and things to consider, but they will also help you reconnect with the glorious, unique character that's been within you all along.

# LOW BATTERY QUESTIONS

1. Let's cover the demographic stuff first. Who does this journal belong to?

   Name: ..............................

   Age: ..............................

   Gender: ..............................

   Hometown: ..............................

   Disability status: ..............................

2. How much do you think your chronic illness influences your identity at the moment?

| Always | Often | Sometimes | Occasionally | Never |
|---|---|---|---|---|
| 1 | 2 | 3 | 4 | 5 |

3. How much would you like your chronic illness to influence your identity? Remember, no incorrect answers here!

| Always | Often | Sometimes | Occasionally | Never |
|---|---|---|---|---|
| 1 | 2 | 3 | 4 | 5 |

4. How would you describe your personality? Circle five to ten words that best describe you.

| | | | |
|---|---|---|---|
| Ambitious | Bright | Calm | Unpredictable |
| Generous | Curious | Dedicated | Benevolent |
| Witty | Loyal | Gentle | Creative |
| Faithful | Outspoken | Quirky | Affectionate |
| Confident | Adventurous | Brave | Kind |

| Conscientious | Empathetic | Spontaneous | Easy-going |
| --- | --- | --- | --- |
| Honest | Optimistic | Aggressive | Sociable |
| Imaginative | Irritable | Charming | Outgoing |

**5.** Rank these values (1–5) in order of their importance to your identity.

| Number (1–5) | Quality |
| --- | --- |
| ○ | Hobbies and interests |
| ○ | Personality characteristics |
| ○ | Demographic factors, e.g. gender, ethnicity, disability status |
| ○ | Values and beliefs about the world |
| ○ | Relationships with others |

COLOURING PAGE »→

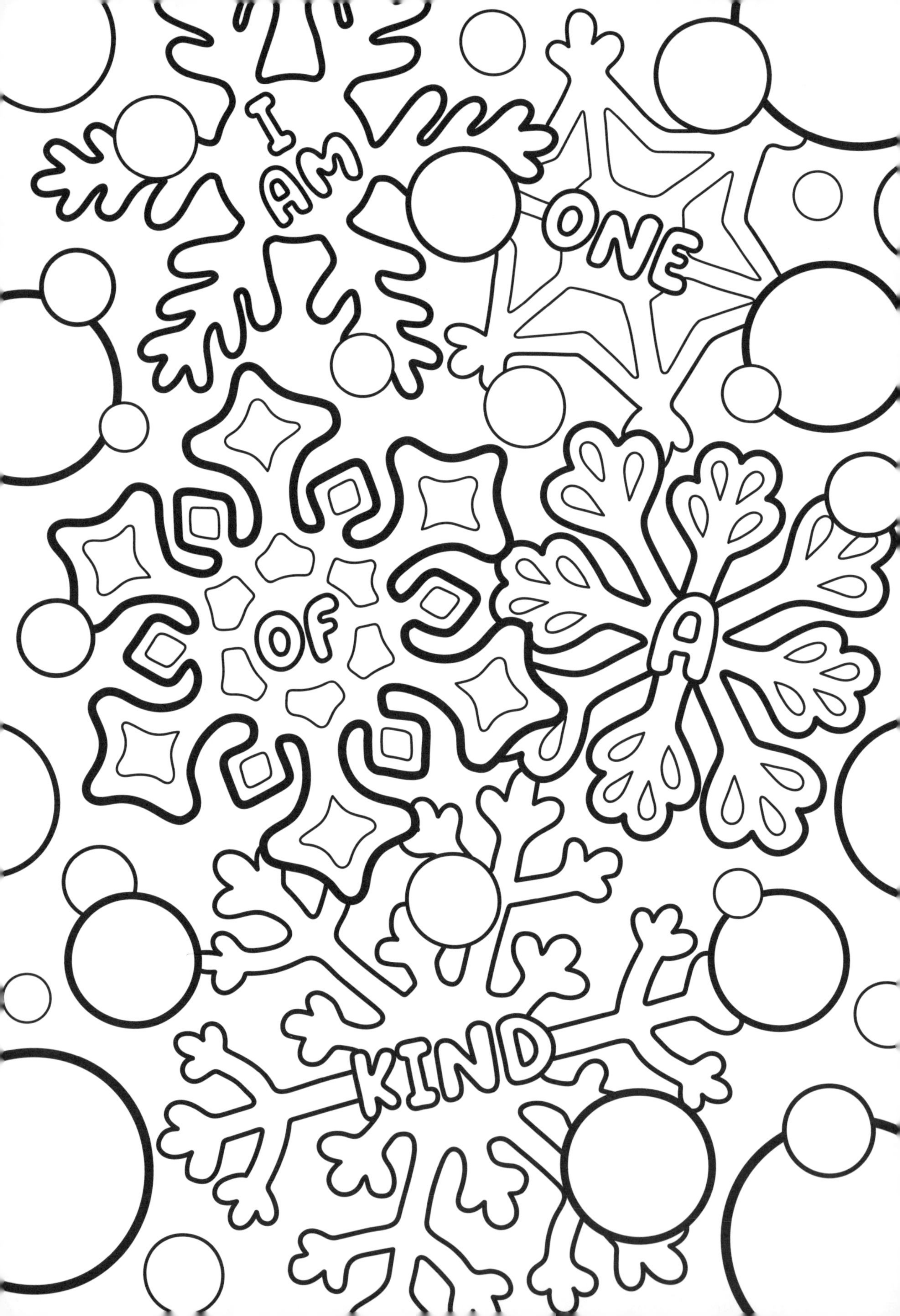
I AM
ONE
OF
A
KIND

# MEDIUM BATTERY QUESTIONS

1. This or that? Circle your favourite answer for each choice, or write your own answer next to it – after all, not everybody fits into one binary.

| | | |
|---|---|---|
| **Introvert** | or | **extravert?** |
| **Morning** | or | **evening?** |
| **Books** | or | **movies?** |
| **Tea** | or | **coffee?** |
| **Films** | or | **TV series?** |
| **Breakfast** | or | **dinner?** |
| **Logic** | or | **emotion?** |
| **Fiction** | or | **non-fiction?** |
| **Cats** | or | **dogs?** |
| **Sweet** | or | **savoury?** |

2. What three words do you think others would use to describe you?

3. These are a few of my favourite things... Circle the activities that make you happy. Not all of these will be accessible for people at different illness severities, so feel free to add in your own answers too.

| | | |
|---|---|---|
| Reading | Colouring in | Watching TV |
| Gaming | Knitting | Watching films |
| Crochet | Crafting | Watching YouTube videos |

(list continues overleaf!)

Musical theatre

Singing

Content creation

Trying new restaurants

Going out for brunch

Cooking

Baking

Scrapbooking

Journaling

Sports or adaptive activities

Shopping

Day trips

Digital drawing

Holidays and adventures

Music

Socialising with friends

Going to pubs or bars

Watching sports

Social media scrolling

Audiobooks

Pottery

Learning a language or skill

Other

..................................

..................................

**4.** Choose your top three hobbies or interests from the answers you have circled above. What is it that you most enjoy about them? Write your answer underneath each one – for example, finding them relaxing, spending time with others, challenging yourself...

1

2

3

**5.** Choose another hobby from the list above that interests you. How might you adapt this hobby to suit your access needs?

6. Picture the adaptations or adjustments that would enable you to enjoy this new activity (including resting and pacing), and draw or doodle them below.

7. Chronic illness can significantly affect who we are as a person. List three ways you think chronic illness has negatively impacted your identity, and three ways chronic illness has positively impacted your identity. Don't worry if this is a struggle to complete right now – you can always return to it later.

| **How chronic illness has negatively impacted my identity,** e.g. being more irritable or insecure | **How chronic illness has positively impacted my identity,** e.g. increasing empathy for others or learning to self-advocate |
|---|---|
| | |
| | |
| | |

**8.** Disability and ableism can also take a toll on our self-esteem, but this doesn't completely eclipse who we are. Use this space to write down or draw at least five of your favourite qualities about yourself.

**9.** If you had a magic potion that could change one thing about the world we live in, what would you choose and why? Write it on the label below!

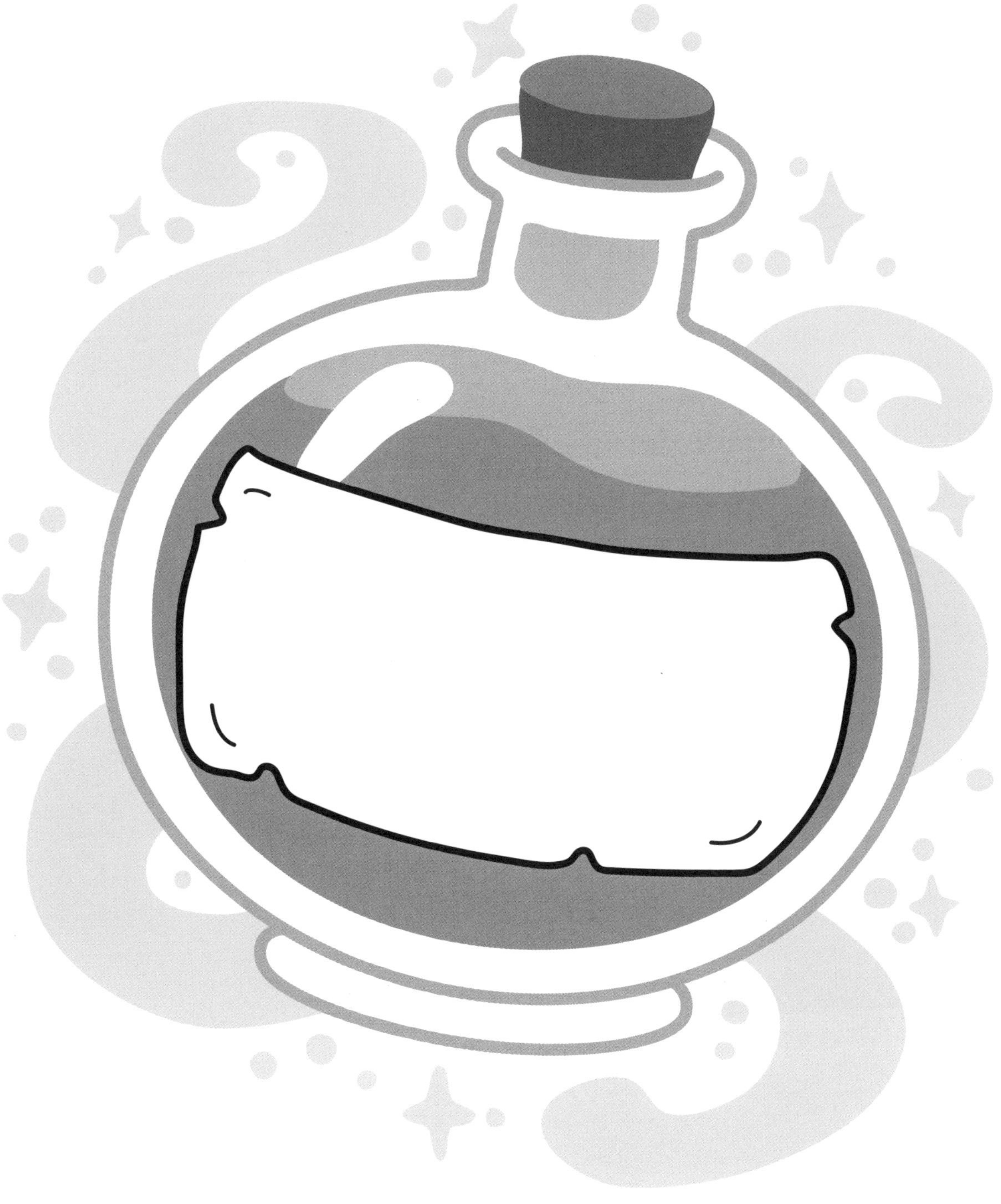

**10.** Word search. Find the following words and phrases associated with identity. Did any of them jump out at you before the others?

| H | R | U | K | U | R | R | T | E | X | X | Y | X | I | S |
|---|---|---|---|---|---|---|---|---|---|---|---|---|---|---|
| Y | O | E | O | K | W | X | B | P | W | C | M | O | N | F |
| O | L | B | W | Y | N | Q | X | Q | Y | X | O | X | Q | M |
| A | E | V | B | O | R | S | Q | B | T | D | N | I | E | T |
| L | V | H | Z | I | P | C | E | W | I | M | O | E | K | G |
| P | A | O | S | C | E | E | Y | P | T | U | T | T | H | W |
| C | L | G | G | P | Z | S | A | D | N | S | U | Z | P | R |
| Z | U | O | Q | Y | T | N | N | N | E | J | A | Q | Z | H |
| J | E | D | V | R | X | K | F | F | D | O | T | F | Z | Y |
| K | S | R | T | D | L | P | L | M | I | Y | M | O | S | Y |
| H | F | K | A | N | L | E | S | S | N | G | E | E | V | S |
| F | I | P | E | R | S | O | N | A | L | I | T | Y | H | V |
| S | C | I | H | P | A | R | G | O | M | E | D | O | N | E |
| S | Q | B | O | N | O | P | X | B | Q | K | T | T | X | D |
| V | I | S | B | R | H | T | D | L | D | H | P | B | J | H |

Identity
Personality
Values
Power
Self-esteem
Hobbies
Demographics
Autonomy

# 'BETTER' BATTERY QUESTIONS

1. Doodle a self-portrait of how you see yourself. Now doodle a self-portrait of how you think others see you. Are there any key differences?

**How I see myself**

**How I think others see me**

**2.** If you wanted to tell somebody else about your chronic illness, how would you explain it to them? Write down your answer in one or two sentences, in this speech bubble.

**3.** Often, we don't give ourselves the time and space to grieve the things we've lost from life due to chronic illness. Similarly, it's not always easy to recognise the ways that chronic illness may have positively influenced our lives too. Use this space to write down some of the things you grieve for, that chronic illness has taken away, and then use the adjoining space to balance these out with things that chronic illness has made you feel grateful for. It's okay if you can't balance out your grief with gratitude right now – life isn't always as balanced as we'd like it to be, and that's totally fine.

| **I grieve for...** | **I'm grateful for...** |
|---|---|
| | |
| | |
| | |

**4.** Some of our personality traits are impacted by chronic illness, while others remain more stable. Look at the words you circled in question three of the low battery questions to describe your identity. On the following diagram, list the traits that you feel are affected by your chronic illness around the edges of the person, and the ones you feel are more stable inside the diagram, at the person's core.

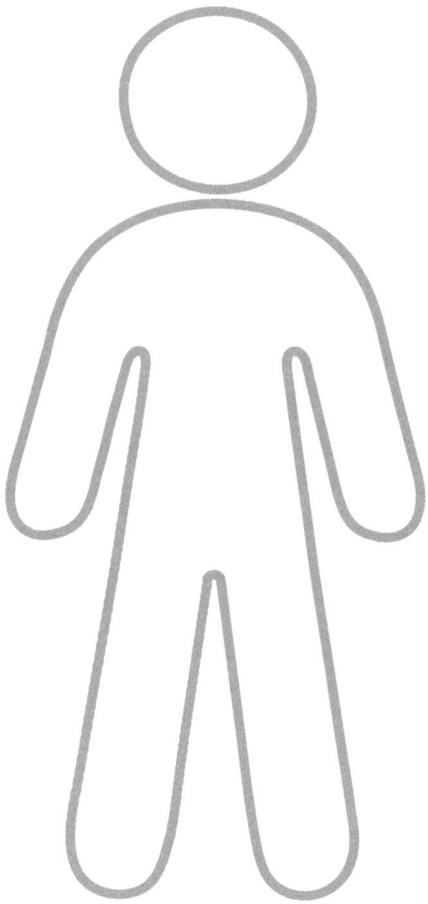

5. **Journal prompt:** Reflect on your current sense of identity, and the answers you have identified in this section.

    - How would you describe your identity at this point in time, and how is this influenced by your health condition?
    - Are there any areas where your identity or sense of self currently feels unclear? How might you reconnect with yourself?
    - Describe the best version of yourself – what does your identity look like in this scenario?

# SECTION 2
# LIFE LOOKS LIKE THIS

NO matter how long you've lived with your chronic illness, the chances are you'll have experienced people trying to 'heal' you or share unsolicited opinions on treatments that might help. Do these people have any medical training or experience that qualifies them to give this advice? Not usually, no. Does that stop them? Still no.

Chronic illness affects all of us uniquely. One style of condition management that helps one person could make zero difference to or even harm another, and vice versa. I believe there's a lot we can learn from each other, and information sharing is a valuable tool, but at the end of the day, we know our individual selves better than anybody. We are the best placed to judge what will or will not help us.

Therefore, the aim of this section is not to try and dispel medical advice or alter any existing treatment plan you have. None of this is a substitute for support or guidance from a medical professional who specialises in your condition, though goodness knows it sometimes feels as if it would be easier to spot a rogue unicorn roaming the town centre than find one of those. Instead, we'll use this section to take a look at the way you currently Do Life. Although we are not personally responsible for our illness trajectory and this is largely out of our control, our lifestyle can have an impact on our health – not only our physical wellbeing but our mental wellbeing too.

Don't worry, I'm not about to morph into one of those personal trainers or nutritionists who lectures you about how there's no excuse for not being active or eating the very specific diet that they're probably paid a commission to recommend. I'm also not going to emulate one of those gurus who encourages you to wake up at 5am and start the day with a solid hour of yoga – these things can be genuinely helpful and enjoyable for some people and we shouldn't minimise that, but for me personally and perhaps you, an hour of movement in the morning would without doubt write off the rest of the day (and probably the following days) before it had even begun.

In fact, a lot of the advice we're often given about health and wellbeing isn't particularly inclusive for people with energy-limiting conditions. And more than that, it can often feel as though there's no choice but to plough all of our mental and physical energy into trying to make physical progress if we want to avoid negative assumptions from others. Sometimes, through no fault of our own, we're made to feel as though spending our limited energy on ourselves or the things that make us happy, instead of our condition management, is 'selfish' or 'a waste'. We're having none of that here, though. Our quality of life is significantly impacted by our physical experience of illness or pain, but it's made up of so much other stuff too. This is a space where your happiness and small moments of joy are a central part of the conversation about your wellbeing too.

With no judgement, we're going to look at the things in your day that serve you well, and the things that perhaps serve you less well. The things that provide mental or physical relief or respite, and the things that don't. Our daily routines often become second nature to us and we wade through them on autopilot, especially when we're experiencing brain fog or cognitive fatigue. But today, let's take a moment to think intentionally about the things we do and how we may (if we choose to) adapt them to create a more positive impact on our mental and physical wellbeing.

## LOW BATTERY QUESTIONS

**1.** How much do you feel your current way of life suits your chronic illness or condition management?

| Not at all | Not very much | I'm not sure | Quite well | Very well |
|---|---|---|---|---|
| 1 | 2 | 3 | 4 | 5 |

**2.** When you think about what you want out of life, which of these words most jump out at you? Think carefully, and circle three to five of the following answers that you value the most highly.

| | |
|---|---|
| Peace | Relaxation |
| New experiences | Achieving goals |
| Mental stimulation | Variety |
| Relationships with others | Stability |
| Solitude | Creativity |

**3.** It's important to recognise that we all have different demands on our time – for example, being in work, requiring frequent hospital visits or treatment regimes, or having parenting or caregiving responsibilities. Based on your current support system and any duties towards others, how much autonomy do you feel you have over your daily routine?

| None at all | Not very much | It depends | A little | A lot |
|---|---|---|---|---|
| 1 | 2 | 3 | 4 | 5 |

4. What is the time of day you most look forward to? Draw or doodle your answer.

COLOURING PAGE →

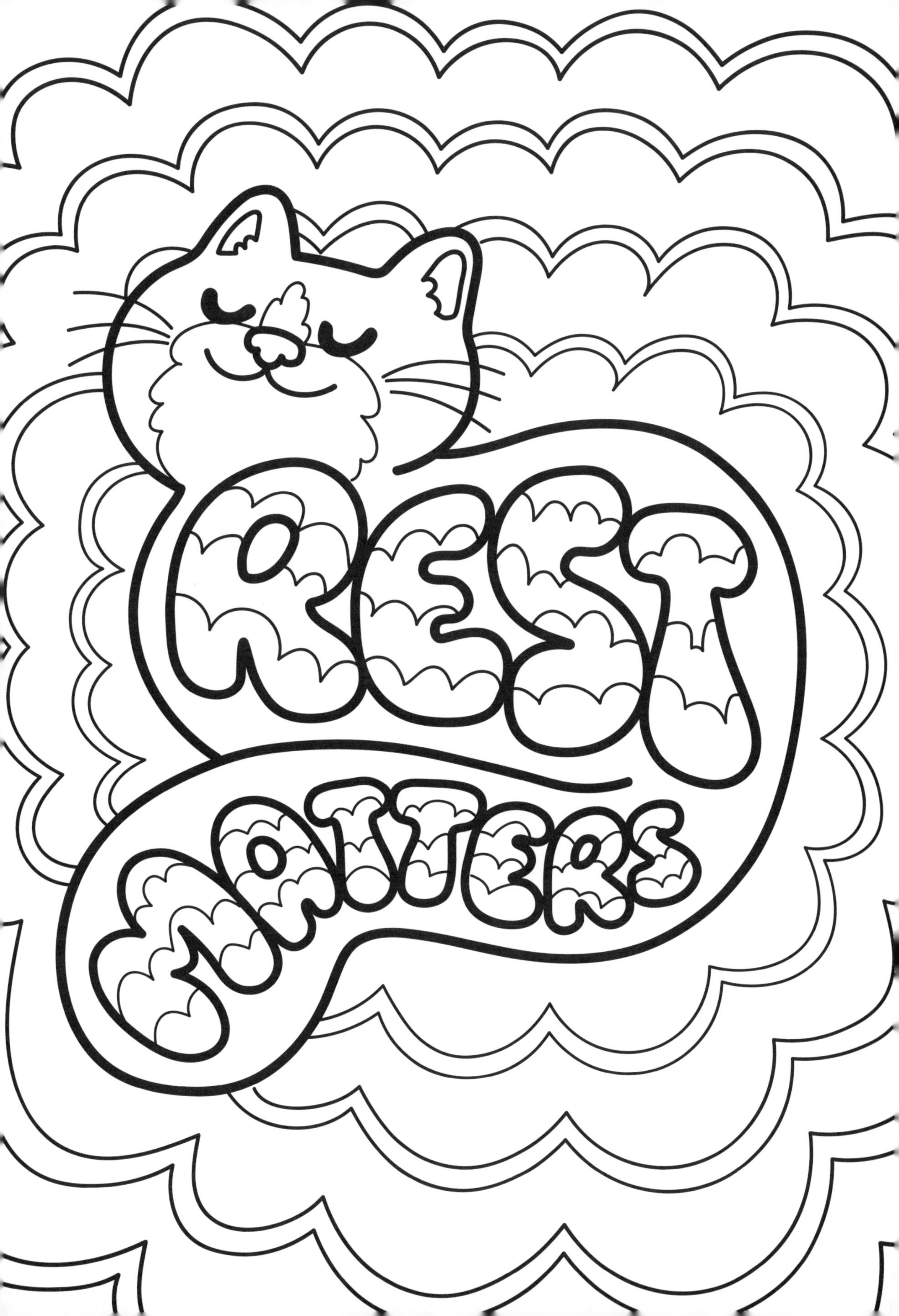
REST
MATTERS

## MEDIUM BATTERY QUESTIONS

If you struggle with disordered eating, please skip ahead to question 5.

**1.** Speaking about food should always be handled sensitively, especially when chronic illness is part of the picture. You may rely on somebody else's cooking if you're not well enough to do it yourself, or have to prioritise easy-to-prepare foods to conserve your energy levels. You may have to follow a special diet for treatment regimes, or you may live with food allergies or intolerances. Even if this is not the case for you, you will probably have noticed that some foods make you feel better than others, and also that some foods bring you more joy than others. Think about the meals you ate yesterday. With no judgement, complete this table.

| **Breakfast** | |
|---|---|
| **Lunch** | |
| **Dinner/Tea** | |
| **Snacks** | |
| **Drinks** | |

If you can, think about how each meal made you feel afterwards. Using three colours or highlighters, go through your responses and identify foods that made you feel good, foods that were neutral or had no noticeable effect, and use another colour for anything that made your symptoms feel worse. How many foods fell into each of these categories?

**2.** Now think only about the foods that bring you joy. Draw or make a list of your favourite meals, drinks, and snacks here.

**3.** With your observations from the above table and incorporating some of your favourite things, draw up a meal plan for the next seven days. Meal planning can feel like such a chore, but planning for the future can save us so much cognitive energy, help us to prepare and pace ourselves more appropriately, and select choices that make us feel at our best.

| | **Breakfast** | **Lunch** | **Dinner/Tea** | **Snacks and drinks** |
|---|---|---|---|---|
| Mon | | | | |
| Tue | | | | |
| Wed | | | | |
| Thu | | | | |
| Fri | | | | |
| Sat | | | | |
| Sun | | | | |

**4.** Nobody knows your body and mind better than you do. You are never obliged to try experimental or alternative treatments to appease others, but you may have tried different kinds of approaches to managing your condition yourself. Use this space to record what you have found helpful or unhelpful. Add the helpful stuff to your backpack as tools to carry with you, put the unhelpful stuff in the bin, and leave the neutral stuff around the edges in case somebody else would like to claim it.

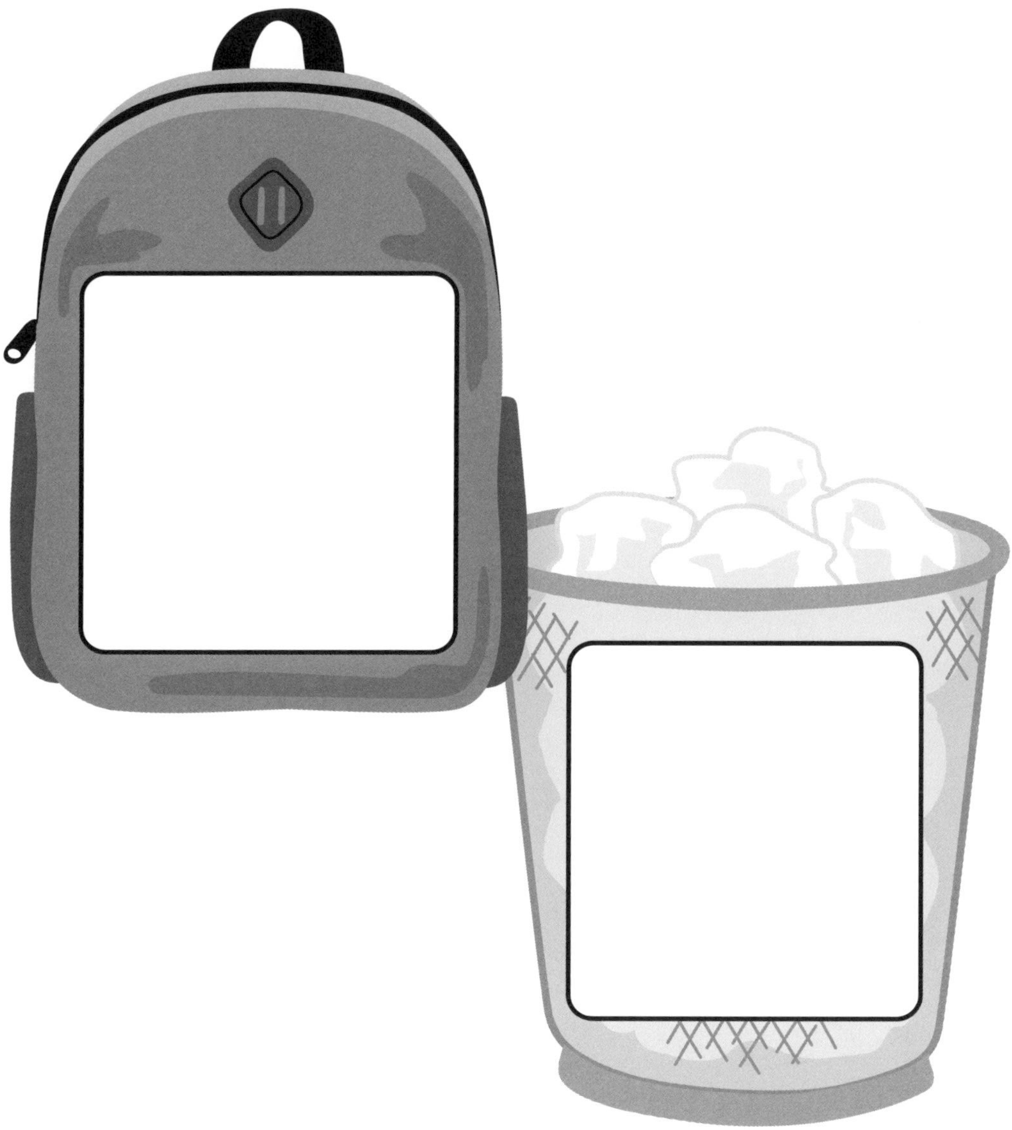

**5.** One of your friends reaches out to you and offers you one unconditional act of kindness to make your day brighter. What do you ask them for?

**6.** Think about the answer you have just identified above. What made you choose it? What does it say about the things that matter to you at this point in your life, and are there any ways you may act on this?

7. This or that? Circle the answer you would most often choose in your daily life...

| | | |
|---|---|---|
| **Slow morning** | or | **get up and go?** |
| **Comfy clothes** | or | **an outfit of your choice?** |
| **To-do list** | or | **go with the flow?** |
| **Time with others** | or | **time to yourself?** |
| **Online connection** | or | **digital detox?** |

8. A good evening routine is the key to the most restful night's sleep possible. Describe or illustrate your current evening routine.

9. We can often meet a lot of internal resistance when we try to make changes to our evening routine, especially when we're dealing with low energy. However, is there anything you would like to change? What could you do to make this change easier for yourself?

## 'BETTER' BATTERY QUESTIONS

**1.** For many of us, our symptoms naturally differ at different time points in a day. For example, some people experience better cognitive function in the morning, while others find this easier during early evening. Some people have fewer debilitating symptoms after they've eaten, compared with how they are when they first wake up.

Using a traffic light system, document your general symptom trajectory (for physical, mental, and emotional energy) over the course of the day in the table below. Colour the box in red if your energy is at its worst at this time, orange if it's around your baseline, or green if this is one of your better points in the day.

| Time of day | Physical energy? | Mental energy? | Emotional energy? |
|---|---|---|---|
| Early morning after waking | | | |
| Mid/late morning | | | |
| Midday | | | |
| Early afternoon | | | |
| Mid/late afternoon | | | |
| Dinnertime/ early evening | | | |
| Mid/late evening | | | |
| Bedtime | | | |

The above activity is inspired by the book *Pace Yourself* by Amy Arthur – an excellent read for anybody who struggles with pacing each day.

2. Now, describe your current daily routine, in as much detail as you can. Write the time of day in the column on the left, and describe your activity in the column on the right. Depending on your illness severity, there may be more boxes here than you need, or fewer – feel free to create your own version if this is the case.

| Time | Activity |
|---|---|
| | |
| | |
| | |
| | |
| | |
| | |
| | |

**3.** Compare the daily routine table you have just completed with the table documenting your patterns of energy over the day. Is there anything you have noticed? Are any of your daily activities ideally placed for the amount of energy you have available at that time, and are there others that might be better if allocated to a different point in time? Are there rest breaks at regular intervals over your day?

**4.** What does rest look like to you? Describe or illustrate your answers below.

**Physical rest**

**Mental rest**

**Emotional rest**

5. **Journal prompt:** Reflect on what life looks like for you right now.

    - Think about your ideal way of life – not necessarily your 'dream life', but a way of existing that is realistic alongside any health constraints or life circumstances. In this ideal picture, are there any key themes or qualities that stand out to you?

- Do you think your current daily routines best serve your physical and mental health? Is there anything you would change?
- What is your relationship with rest? Do you think there is enough rest and respite in your current way of life, and if not, how might you create space for more?

# SECTION 3
# BE YOUR OWN HERO

BEING a chronically ill person in an ableist world is tough. Change is happening and the disability movement is gaining traction, but there are still many physical, societal, and systemic barriers we may encounter along the way. As much as I wish it weren't the case, being able to self-advocate and build up your resilience to deal with these challenges is a very important skill – especially as these things definitely don't come easy to all of us.

I'm not a very assertive person by nature. I'm a people-pleaser through and through, and as I've grown older and (somewhat) wiser, this element of my identity has gone from being something I like about myself to something I wish I could change. There is nothing fundamentally wrong with wanting to be liked and held in positive regard by others, but it can make it difficult to set important boundaries that serve our mental and physical wellbeing. For a long time, I would often make myself more unwell than I needed to, rather than run the risk of causing discomfort for others, but I can tell you with complete conviction that this really isn't a sustainable way to live your life. Who would have thought it?

There are some incredible voices in the disability and chronic illness community. People who are absolute powerhouses, using their online platforms to highlight inequalities and call out ableism as and when they encounter it. Often, I wish I could be more like them. I used to beat myself up for not being louder or more outspoken, for shrinking away from conflict rather than standing my ground. However, now I like to look at things in a more balanced way. If you're able to lean into advocating for yourself and others and you're not afraid to use your voice, all power to you. On the other hand, if you find these things more difficult or don't know where to start, I hope you will get a lot of value out of this section.

Self-advocacy is defined as the action of representing yourself, or your views or interests. Sometimes it means challenging injustice, sometimes it's necessary to access the support and adjustments we require, and sometimes it means calling out prejudice in the name of being treated in the same way as others. It's also important to recognise that people who belong to more than one marginalised group, such as being BIPOC (Black, Indigenous, and people of colour) or LGBTQ+ (lesbian, gay, bisexual, transgender, queer or questioning) as well as being chronically ill, have the additional challenge of advocating for and taking care of themselves in a way that accommodates more than one set of social barriers.

When you have a long-term health condition, there are many times when you need to be your own hero. Gaps in social support and widespread disability discrimination in the world around us mean there is often no choice but to stand up for ourselves and fight for what we need. And even if that feels totally impossible for you right now, as it once did for me, I want you to know that you can do this. The more skilled we become at self-advocating, and the better able we are to redefine this and find the communication methods that best suit us, the closer we can get to leading the life we choose.

I've come to learn that you don't always have to be the loudest voice in the room to facilitate change or do what's right for you. In fact, many of the ways we traditionally think about self-advocating may feel so unnatural to you that they drain your precious mental and physical energy and leave you exhausted. This is what we want to avoid. Instead, let's take some time to think about the social issues that matter to you, any barriers or ableism you're contending with at the moment, and what kind of self-advocacy strategies might serve you best.

## LOW BATTERY QUESTIONS

**1.** How would you rate your self-advocacy skills at the moment?

| Non-existent | Not very strong | Moderate | Fairly good | Very good |
|---|---|---|---|---|
| 1 | 2 | 3 | 4 | 5 |

**2.** What are your preferred communication styles when dealing with difficult conversations? Circle three to five phrases that resonate with you from the following list.

Open conversations

Digital communications (e.g. email or social media)

Challenging injustice

Reacting in the moment

Needing time to process before taking action

Handling things independently

Requiring peer support from others

Educating others in person

Educating others online

Empowered by self-advocating

Drained by self-advocating

**3.** Self-confidence can enable self-advocacy. How would you rate your self-confidence at the moment?

| Non-existent | Quite low | Neither high nor low | A work in progress | Very strong |
|---|---|---|---|---|
| 1 | 2 | 3 | 4 | 5 |

4. Think about a time when you felt empowered. Describe or doodle that scenario here.

COLOURING PAGE »→

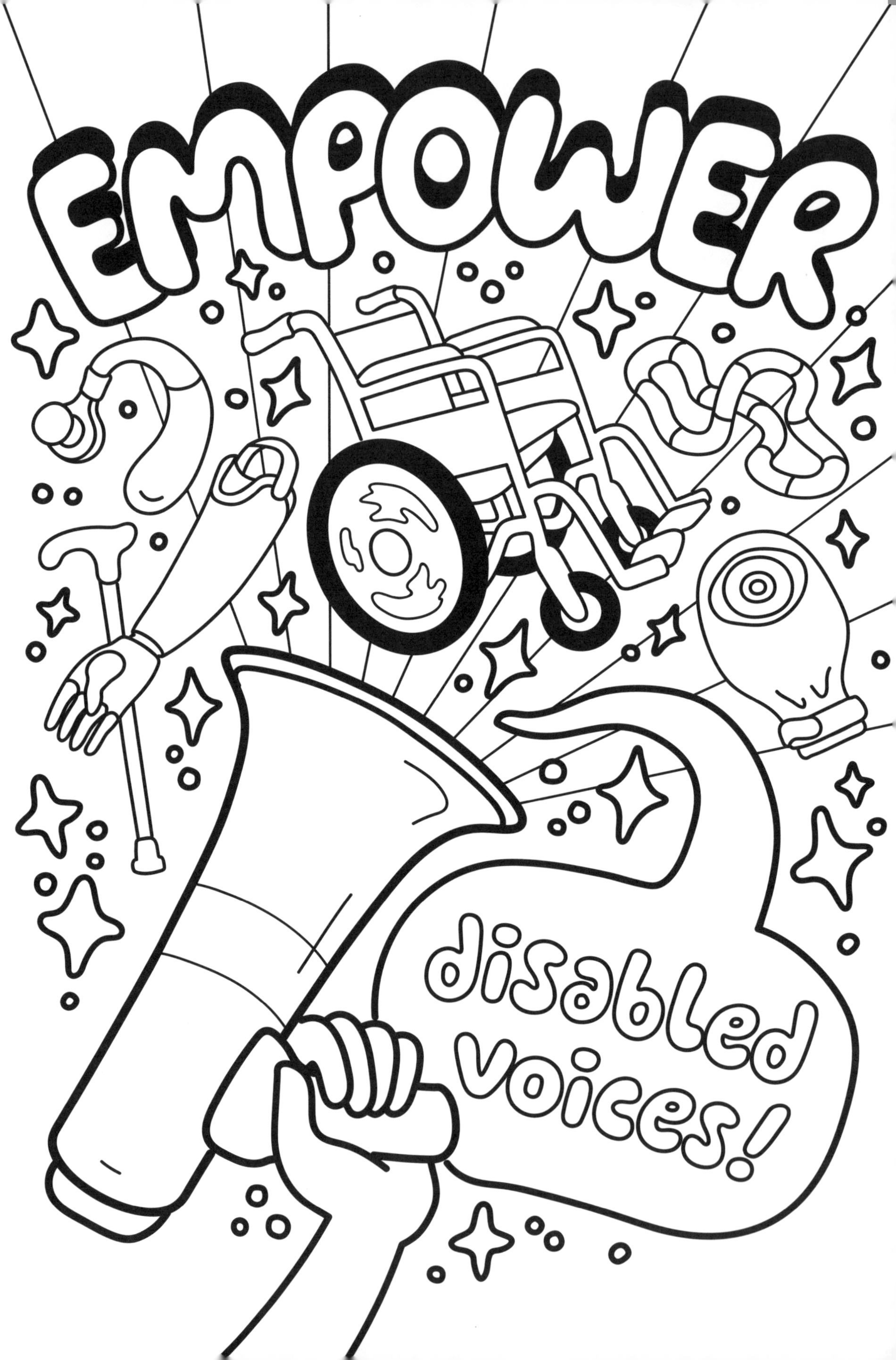
EMPOWER
disabled voices!

## MEDIUM BATTERY QUESTIONS

1. If you have a more visible disability or use mobility aids, you might have been asked invasive questions about your condition by strangers in the world around you. Whether or not you answer or disclose your disability is entirely up to you, but it can be helpful to have a go-to answer in the back of your mind to save you cognitive energy in the moment. If somebody asks you about your condition and you don't want to further the conversation, what might you say back to them?

**If they say...**

**Then I could say...**

2. Think about a time when you had a negative experience of self-advocacy – for example, not getting the outcome you had hoped for or coming away feeling drained or defeated. Describe the situation, and your response, below.

3. How did you feel after this scenario had taken place? From the list of emotions below, circle the ones that apply to you.

| | | | |
|---|---|---|---|
| Empowered | Heard/Listened To | Drained | Proud |
| Angered | Validated | Insecure | Lonely |

4. Consider the emotions you've chosen above. Are you surprised by any of them? Do you think any were influenced by your choice of communication style?

5. We are not responsible for other people's outcomes or ableism in the world around us, but is there anything you would choose to do differently if you were in this situation again?

**6.** If you can, think about a time when you had a positive experience of self-advocacy – for example, facilitating a positive interaction or response or coming away feeling as if you had gone about things in a way that was accessible for you. If you can't think of one, imagine one you might encounter in the future. Describe the situation, and your response, below.

7. How did you feel after this scenario had taken place? Colour in the mood faces that apply to you.

Empowered

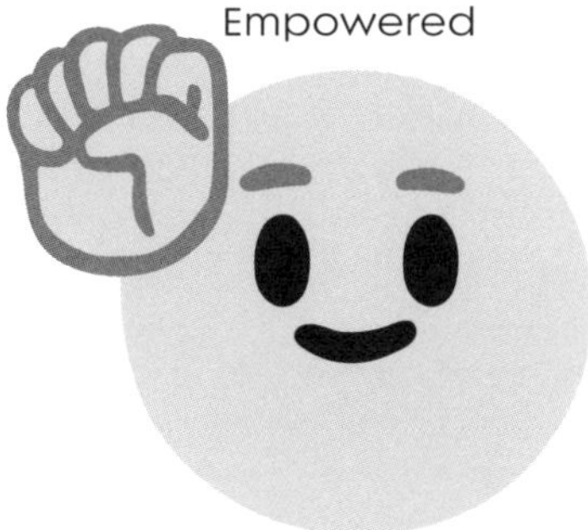

Angered

Heard/Listened To

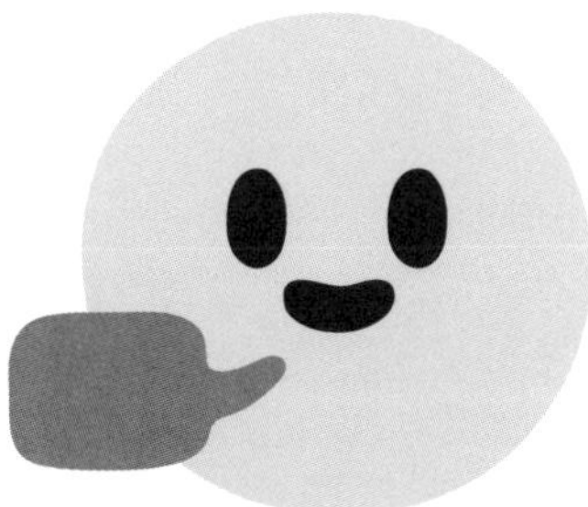

Validated

Drained

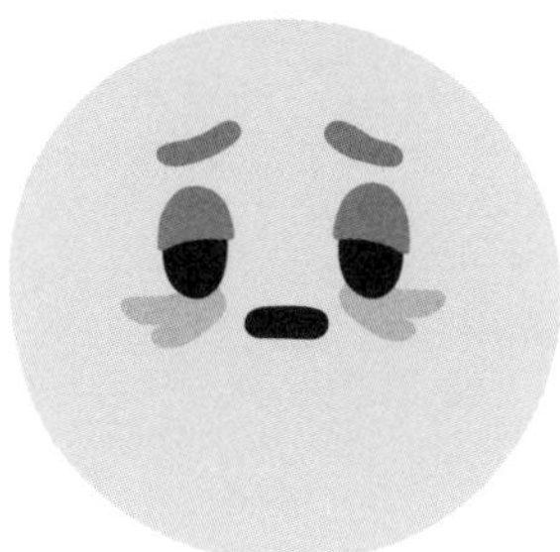

Insecure

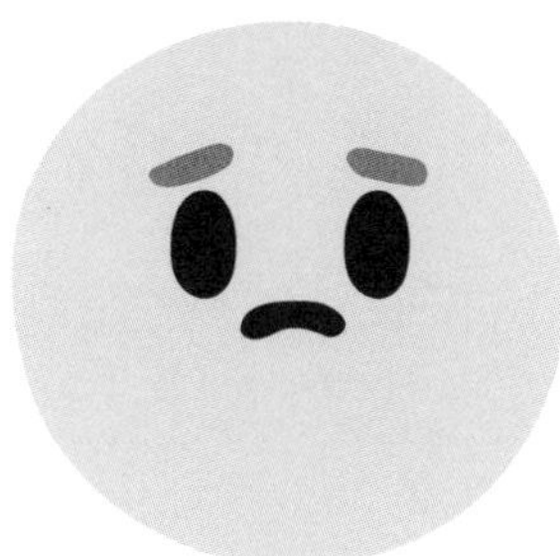

Proud

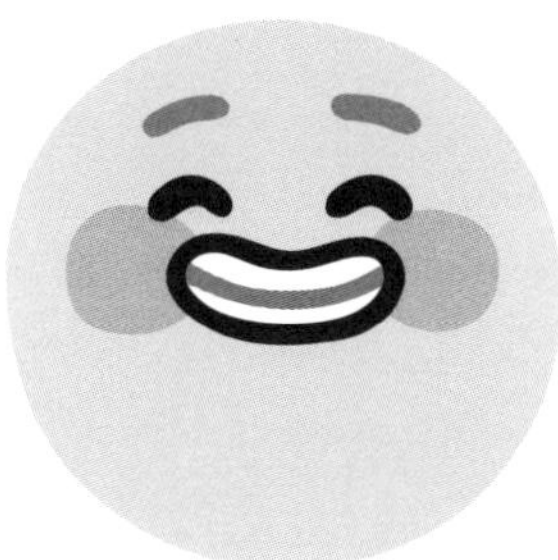

Lonely

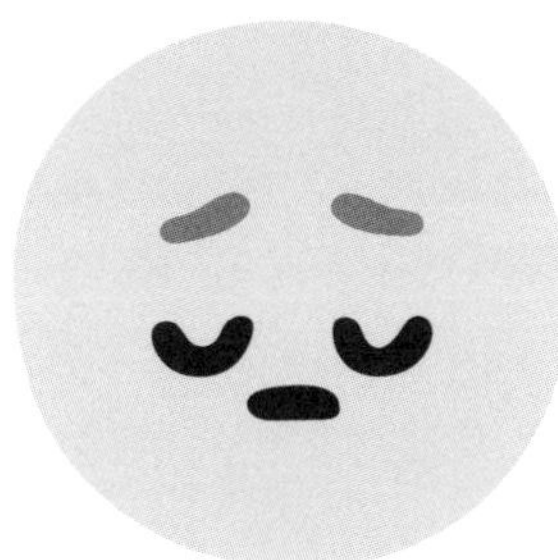

**8.** Consider the emotions you've chosen above. Are you surprised by any of them? Can you attribute any of them to specific moments during your experience?

**9.** Sometimes we can do everything right and still not be treated the way we should be. However, can you identify anything about this interaction that might have led to the positive experience you had?

**10.** We all have qualities that make us capable self-advocates, even qualities we might not typically associate with this skill. Some of mine include being able to see things from somebody else's point of view, being knowledgeable about disability rights, and knowing when to walk away. Annotate this diagram with some of your own skills that make you capable of self-advocacy – there will probably be far more than you originally thought.

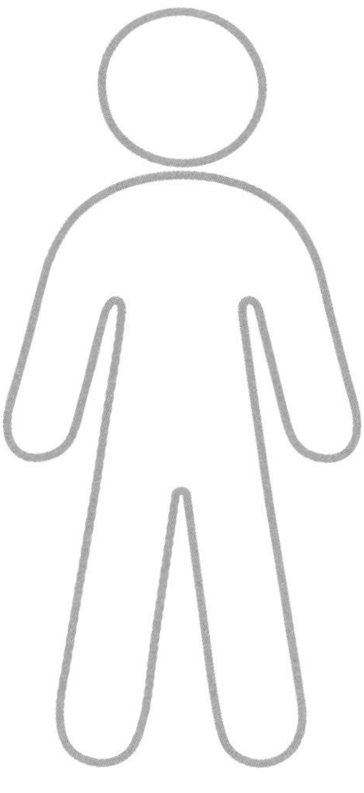

# 'BETTER' BATTERY QUESTIONS

1. Sometimes difficult situations are worth using exertion to resolve, and sometimes it's better to hold on to your precious energy and walk away. Think about the stakes below, and use symbols or colour coding to indicate which of the outcomes feel 'worth the energy' to justify challenging them.

| **Situation** | **Worth your energy?** |
|---|---|
| An anonymous stranger leaves a derogatory comment on social media | |
| A friend makes an incorrect assumption about your condition | |
| A stranger tuts at you for using the priority seat on public transport | |
| You are not offered reasonable adjustments during a job interview | |
| Somebody asks, 'What's wrong with you?' when you're using mobility aids | |
| A family member offers unsolicited advice on your condition management | |
| A shop assistant speaks to the person you're with rather than you | |
| A medical professional trivialises your condition or symptoms | |

2. You've received an email from somebody newly diagnosed with the same chronic illness as you. They are feeling worried about the challenges ahead of them and how to stand up for themselves when times are tough. How would you reply? Write your response below, including any tips or advice you would share.

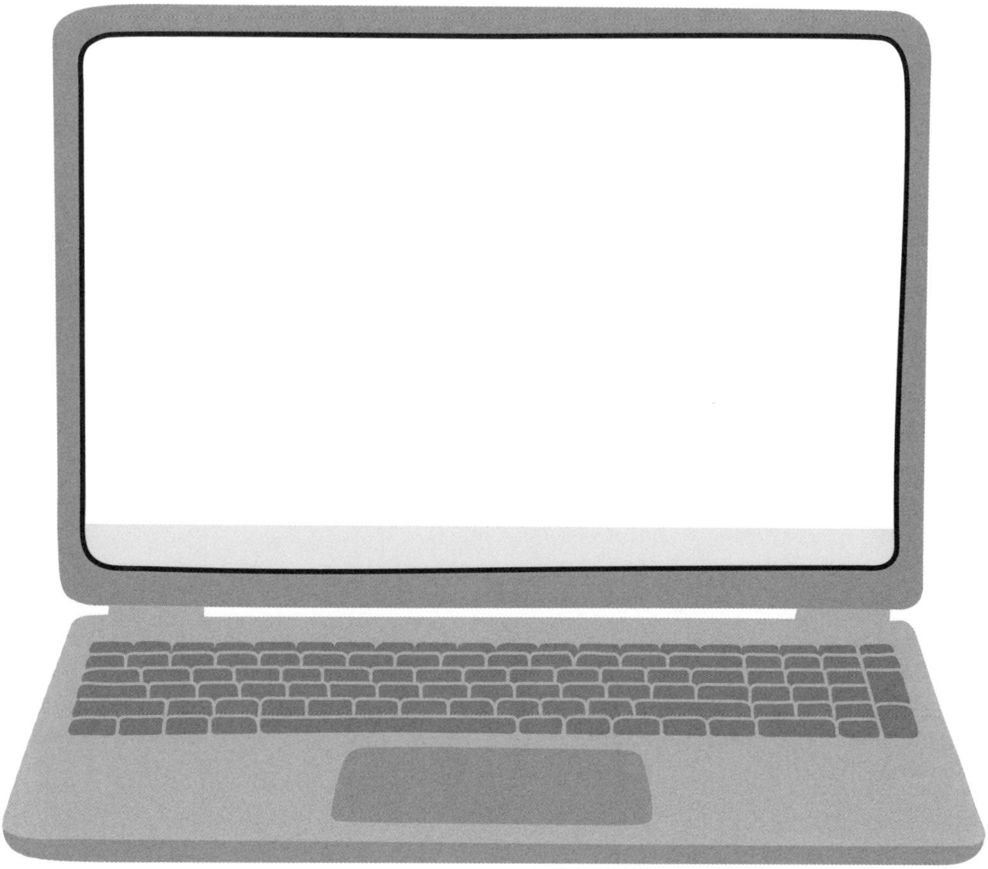

**3.** It's impossible to predict the future, but are there any barriers you are likely to encounter in the coming days, weeks, or months where you may need to self-advocate? How might you deal with them?

| Situation | How might you respond? |
|---|---|
| | |
| | |
| | |
| | |
| | |

**4.** Self-advocacy isn't all doom and gloom, and it doesn't always have to feel like self-defence. When you manage to educate somebody or have an everyday conversation that leads to positive change, it can be one of the best feelings in the world. When you self-advocate, what do you hope to achieve for yourself and/or others? How would you like to feel after an interaction when you've self-advocated?

5. **Journal prompt:** What does self-advocacy look like for you?

- What are your preferred communication styles when dealing with tricky situations? Do you prefer to hash things out in the moment or walk away and reflect before using your voice?
- Is there anything that holds you back from self-advocating at the moment? Why do you think this is?
- How will you be your own hero in the future, in a way that's harmonious with your physical and mental health needs?

# TIME CAPSULE 2

Use this space to record information about you, your chronic illness, and your health and wellbeing at this moment in time. You'll have the opportunity to do this throughout the book, so you can keep in tune with how your thoughts or feelings are evolving.

**What is the date and time?**

**How is your physical health today?**

**How is your mental health today?**

**What are three things you feel grateful for today?**

**What challenges are you facing at the moment?**

**Time to thought-dump. What's on your mind today?**

SECTION 4

# CREATE YOUR HAPPY PLACE

WHEN you're first becoming acquainted with a chronic illness, it can feel all-consuming. Regardless of whether the onset of your condition was slow or sudden, it can be a real shock to the system. Right now, it may feel as though it's taking everything you have simply to get through the day. When you're living with an energy impairment, it often feels as if your usable hours are totally gobbled up by the tasks that are necessary for survival, with hardly anything left to spare.

During the first few years of my chronic illness, I resented the idea that I had any control over my happiness while living this way. How could I possibly add more joy into my life when some days I could barely put one foot in front of the other?

Before this point, I had constantly been chasing the highs in life – filling each day with activities and social gatherings, collecting accomplishments, and making grand plans for the future. I always admired people who were able to take things at a slower pace and appreciate the little things in life, especially as I believed that I just wasn't wired to be that kind of person myself. Thankfully, I know now that it really is possible to find the good in almost any given moment or day. And most importantly, I know that finding and enjoying the good stuff doesn't negate any of the difficult stuff you may be facing at the same time.

Truthfully, opening my eyes to what might be possible required serious patience – not just from me, but from the people around me too. After all, you can't just *decide* that you want to be happy and totally accepting of the situation – the last thing you want to do is force yourself into a mindset of toxic positivity when deep down you're hurting more than ever before. However, there are many small and accessible ways we might introduce more joy into our daily routines and surroundings. And trust me when I say that sometimes even the tiniest things can bring about an unexpected sense of contentment and wellbeing.

First, we'll consider the things that make your heart happy and make you feel most like yourself. Once we've identified those, we'll consider how we might adapt them, so they can take more of a lead role in your current way of life.

The key thing to remember as you explore this section is that happiness is an abstract concept, and it will always mean different things for different people – we'll use the term 'your happy place' to summarise this concept. We'll look at your current environment, including your surroundings and how you like to fill your time, and consider whether these things currently reflect what you see as your ideal way of life. It can be easy to get carried away with this idea – goodness, just imagine how much of an idyllic rest space we could each create if there was an endless pot of money at our disposal! But what we want to do instead is think about realistic, accessible, and actionable changes we can make to bring us closer to our ideals.

Because of the deep-rooted stigma in society that we have grown up with, many of us (myself included) hold a great deal of internalised ableism, and often we're not even aware of how much it can influence our decision making. You may have been conditioned to believe your needs, and moreover your happiness, matter a little less than everybody else's, simply because you have a long-term condition. I cannot tell you strongly enough how incorrect this is. Your life, your comfort, and your happiness matter enormously. Together, let's begin to reclaim it for ourselves.

# LOW BATTERY QUESTIONS

**1.** Which of these things are most important to your level of daily contentment? Label them 1–5, with 1 being the most important.

- ◯ Comfortable surroundings
- ◯ Favourite possessions
- ◯ Time with family and friends
- ◯ Hobbies and interests
- ◯ Escapism and switch-off time

**2.** This or that? Let's think about your environment – the place, room, or bed where you spend most of your day. Circle the phrases in the following list of different environments that most resonate with you.

**Colourful** or **natural?**

**Minimalist** or **grand?**

**Natural light** or **brightness you can control?**

**Background noise** or **peace and quiet?**

**Escapism** or **being at the heart of the action?**

**Plenty to do** or **no distractions?**

**Favourite scents in the air** or **neutral?**

**Encouraging movement** or **welcoming stillness?**

**Photos of loved ones** or **pinboard of future plans?**

**Nods to nature** or **a safe indoor haven?**

**3.** If you had to choose three words to describe your ideal happy place, what would they be?

**4.** How much do you feel your current environment reflects your ideal happy place?

| Very much | Quite a lot | Somewhat | Not very much | Not at all |
|---|---|---|---|---|
| 1 | 2 | 3 | 4 | 5 |

**COLOURING PAGE** »→

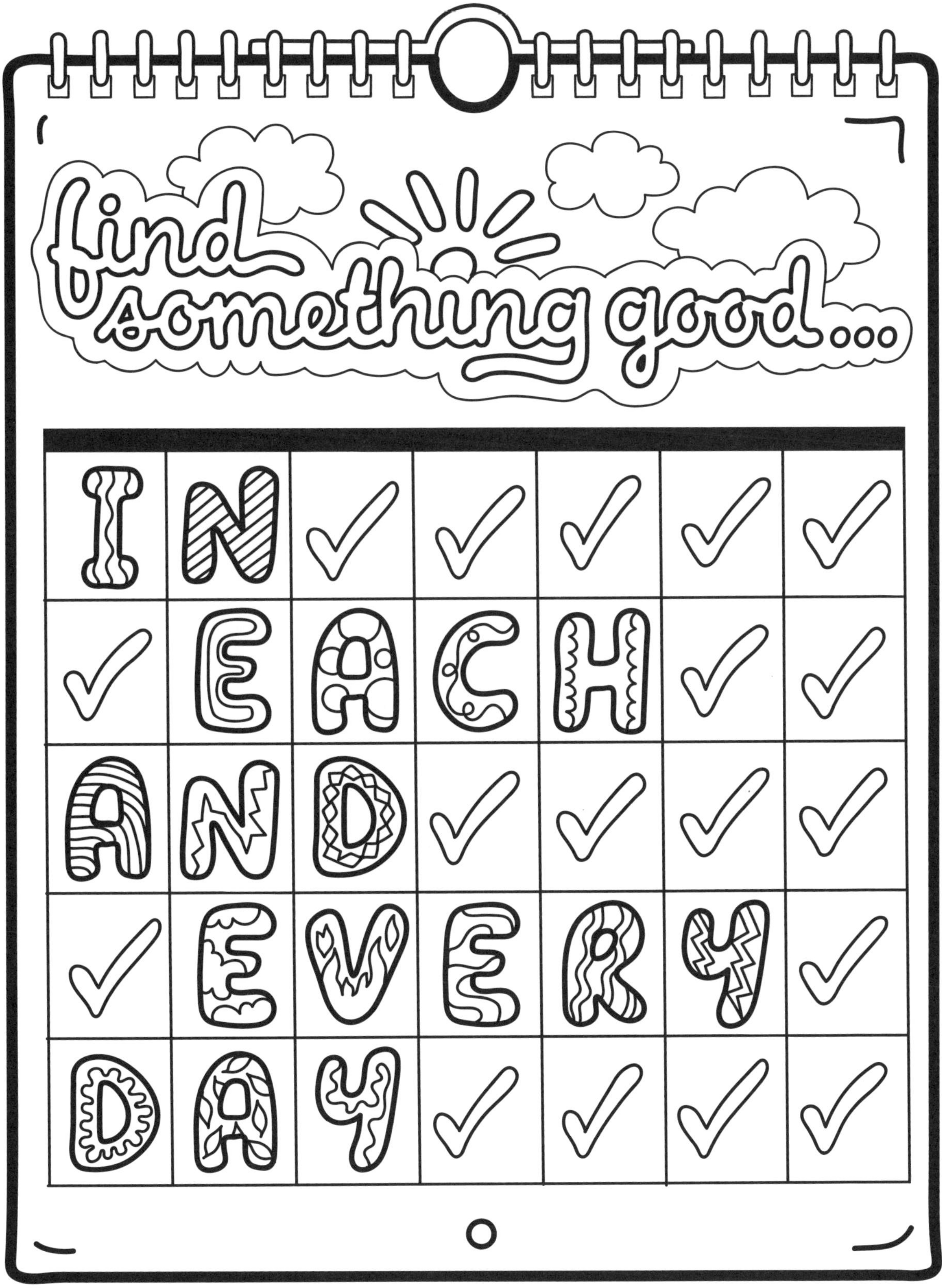
find something good...
IN
EACH
AND
EVERY
DAY

## MEDIUM BATTERY QUESTIONS

1. Energy permitting, think about your favourite things to do. They don't have to be formal hobbies like the ones we considered in Section 1, but simply things you enjoy or look forward to during a typical day (e.g. drinking a morning cup of tea or watching your favourite series). Write down or doodle your top five below.

**2.** Now rank those hobbies according to the ones requiring the least energy to the most energy. Doing this might help you to incorporate them more often into your life, in a way that accommodates fluctuating symptoms and the need for pacing.

1 (uses least energy) ______________________

2 ______________________

3 ______________________

4 ______________________

5 (uses most energy)

**3.** Look around your current environment. If you had to pick your top three favourite possessions, what would you choose? Write or draw your answer below!

4. What made you choose those possessions? What impact do they have on the space you're in?

**5.** Pyjama days are a staple way of life for us chronically ill folk. Use the outline below to design your dream pyjamas or sleepwear.

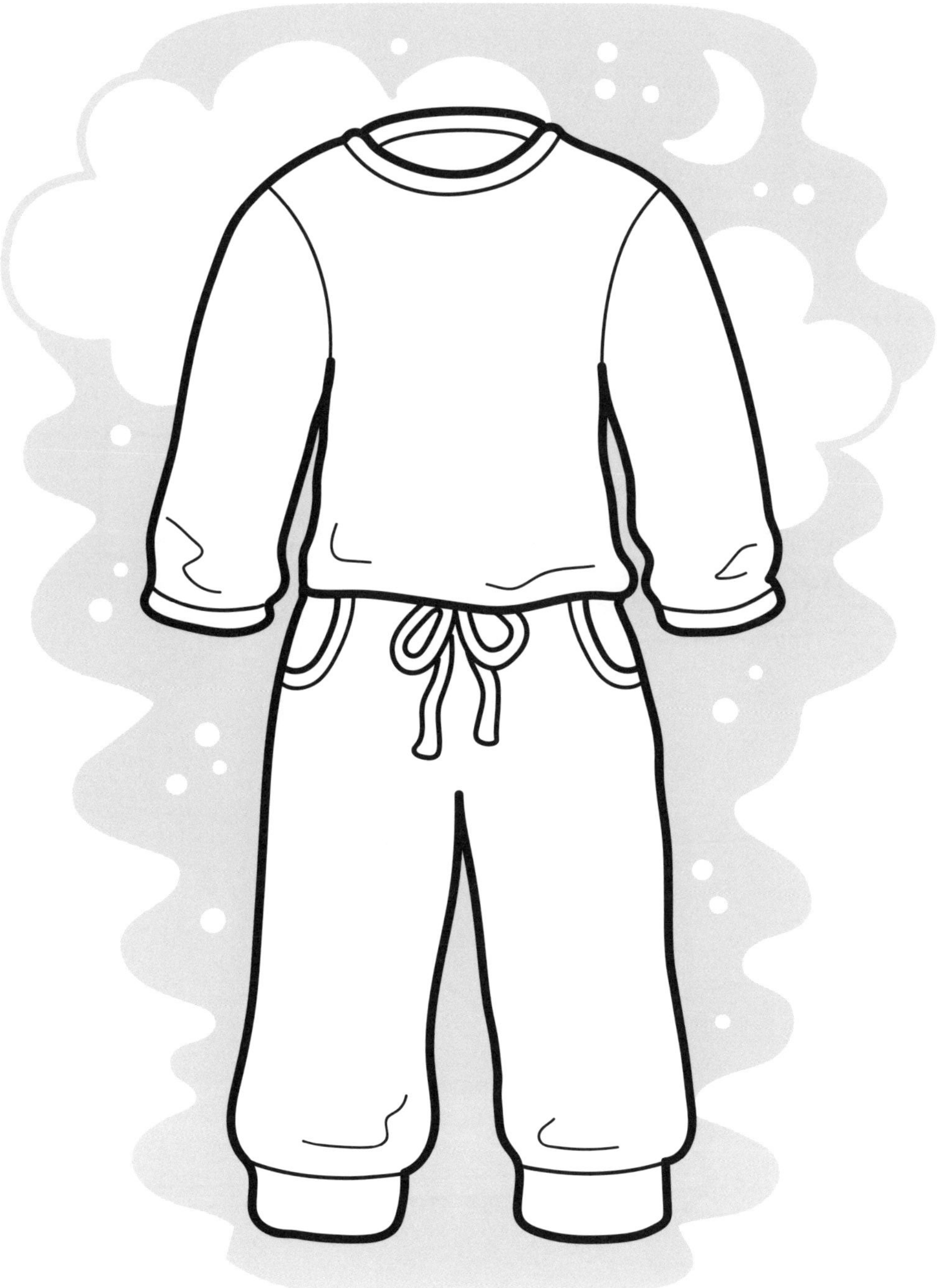

**6.** Resting and/or spending time in bed is also a necessary part of the lifestyle. Use the outline below to design your dream bedding and sleep environment.

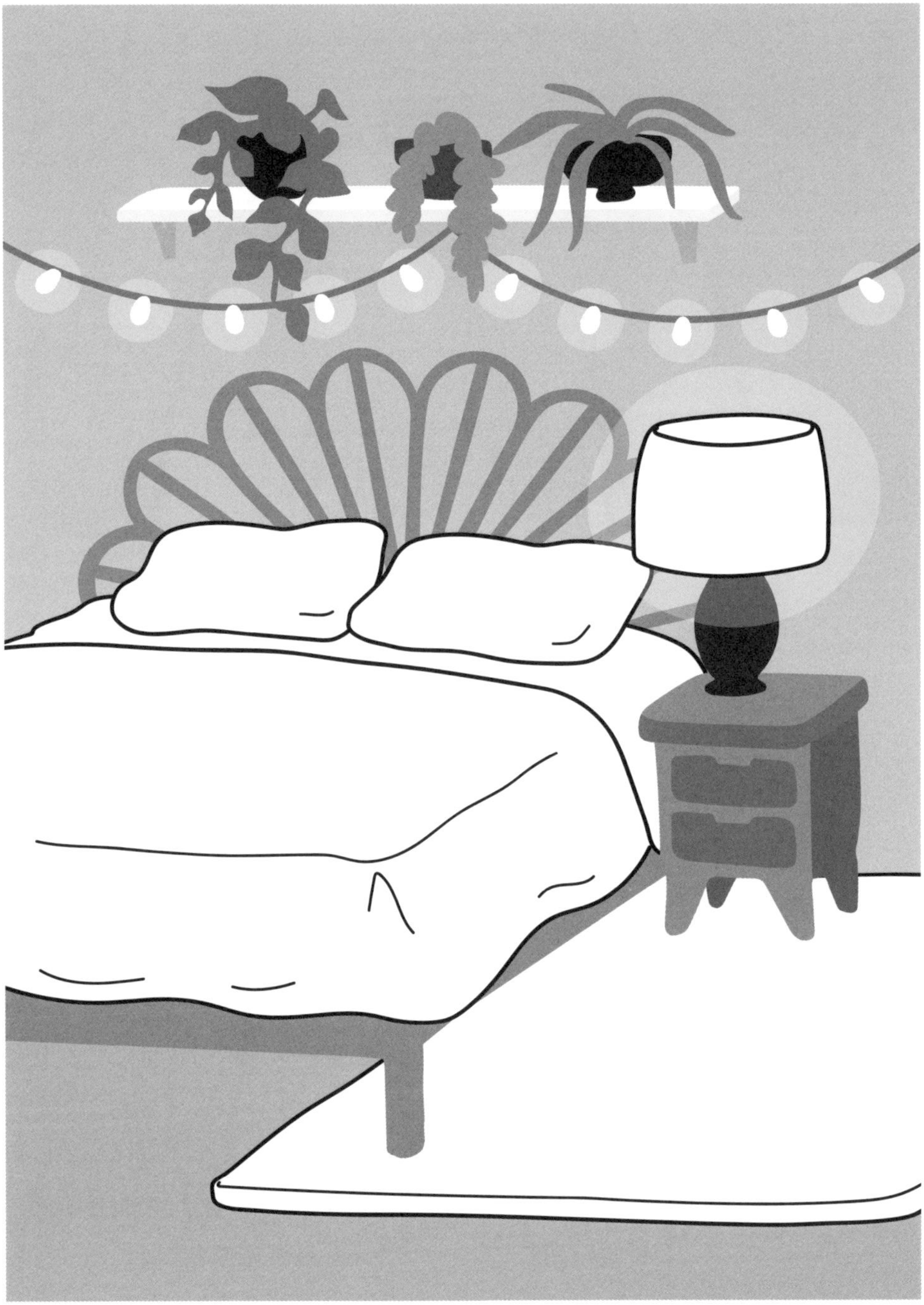

**7.** When you're in bed or resting, what is within your eyeline? What can you see, and does this form part of your happy place? If nothing comes to mind, circle any of the options below that might appeal to you, and consider if/how you could action them.

Photos of loved ones

Favourite quotes

Ceiling stickers or decorations (e.g. glow-in-the-dark stars)

Scenic images of favourite places

Calendar or wall planner sharing things to look forward to

Starry night light projector

A window to see the outdoors

A door to see what's happening elsewhere

**8.** On tougher symptom days, it can be valuable to have a 'chronic illness survival kit' within easy reach – for example, in a drawer in your bed-side table. This kit could contain things that help with your symptoms, items that bring you comfort, treats to make you smile, and so much more. Use this space to write down or doodle what your chronic illness survival kit would contain.

9. Comfort content is so important. What programmes, series, or movies do you turn to when you need relaxation or escapism? Are there any books or podcasts that have a similar effect on you?

10. Think about all of the ideals you have outlined in your answers above. Which of these could you implement in your life, if you choose to? Write down an accessible plan or to-do list for making these things a reality. Don't forget to break tasks down into smaller components and schedule regular rest breaks to aid pacing!

**Happy Place Official Plan of Action**

## 'BETTER' BATTERY QUESTIONS

1. Even if you don't routinely leave the house or you're not hugely into fashion, the way we dress and present ourselves can also bring us joy. Which of your outfits (including pyjamas and comfies, of course!) make you feel most like yourself? Describe or draw them below.

**2.** If you were to create a playlist that captured the essence of your happy place, what songs would it include?

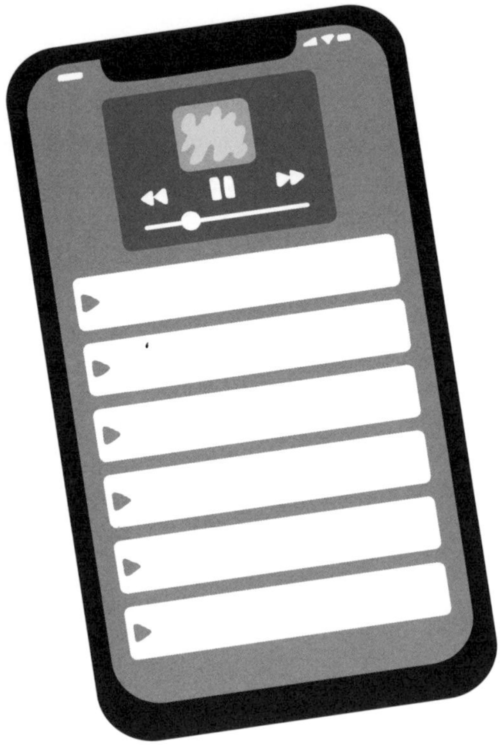

**3.** Being honest with yourself, how much of your daily usable energy do you spend doing things you feel that you *have* to do, versus things you *want* to do?* Mark your answer on the sliding scale below.

**0%** — I spend no energy on the things I want to do

**100%** — I spend all my energy on the things I want to do

*Your response here will, of course, be influenced by your illness severity, responsibilities towards others, and any additional privileges/marginalisation you face. Nobody can realistically spend 100% of their energy the way they want to, but internalised ableism means we often hold ourselves back from prioritising our own happiness. This activity is designed to make you think about the energy you do have at your disposal and how often you 'allow' yourself to spend it on the things that bring you joy.

4. Use the table below to describe a dream day for your future self. Once you've planned it, pick a future date in your calendar and make it a reality!

| **Activity/activities I'd like to do** | **Favourite food, drink, or snacks to accompany plans** | **Solo date or invite others to join?** |
|---|---|---|
| | | |

| **How I'll pace myself** | **Any other access needs to accommodate** | **How I'd like to feel during/ after the day** |
|---|---|---|
| | | |

**5. Journal prompt:** What does your happy place look like for you?

- How close is your current way of life to the way you would like to live? Besides your health condition, is there anything that holds you back from prioritising the things that make you happy?
- Picture and describe an environment you think will best accommodate your chronic illness and also make you feel most like *you*. What can you see, hear, and touch?
- Thinking about your responses to the questions in this section, how might you introduce more joy into your current way of life? Does any element jump out at you more than the others?

## SECTION 5
# YOUR SOCIAL CIRCLE

SPENDING time with your favourite humans is such a gift. However, the challenges of energy-limiting conditions can make it more difficult to meet new people and maintain strong relationships with your existing social circle. As with many elements of life as a chronically ill person, you may be trying to resist this change with all your might. Even if your daily routines have completely shifted to accommodate your condition, you may still be feeling pressure to appear to your nearest and dearest as exactly the same person you were before.

It's human instinct to minimise our struggles sometimes, but I want you to remember that feeling as if your friendships are changing isn't necessarily a bad thing – and it definitely isn't a failure of yours. Yes, there may be people who leave or those you drift away from, or people who you decide to distance yourself from for your own wellbeing. If they can't appreciate the person you are or they're not willing to hold space for your access needs, then that's their loss. However, there can and will be people in your life who love and treasure the whole of you – wonky body and all. Most of us have no real understanding of chronic illness until it happens to us or a loved one. Sometimes, friends just need a little guidance on how they can be what you need them to be.

Even the strongest, longest-term friendships evolve over time. Life happens, and we're constantly changing our social patterns and behaviour. Just as friendships can change when people move away, meet a partner, or become parents, friendships can also change when energy-limiting conditions make themselves known. The secret to holding on to your favourite humans comes from each of you being open and ready to adapt to this change. Through this section, we'll explore how we can gently nudge this evolution into a positive experience: one that not only sidesteps potential hostility but leaves you feeling closer to your loved ones than ever before.

Alternatively, you may be reading this section while struggling with intense feelings of loneliness or isolation. It may be that you don't have a circle of friends around you at the moment, or you feel distant or excluded from the ones you once found comfort in. Perhaps the severity of your condition affects how often you can see or talk to others, or whether you can see or talk to them at all. The loneliness that comes from long-term illness can be crushing, and once it gets hold of you, it can be very difficult to picture things ever being different. But trust me, things can change more than you ever thought possible. During my early twenties, I was surrounded by people but had never felt so lonely. Fast-forward almost a decade and I spend only a fraction of that time around friends now, and yet I feel much more loved and supported than I ever did back then.

When you're ready for it, I promise you there are great people out there who would love to have you in their life. And why wouldn't they, you fabulous thing? Through this section, we'll identify what you truly want out of your friendships and how to make that happen, any insecurities you have around spending time with others, and your boundaries and preferred ways of coping with any difficulties. Let's do this.

## LOW BATTERY QUESTIONS

1. First, let's identify your closest friend or core group of friends who you'll keep in mind while answering these questions – they can be in-person or online friends, or people you've met under any circumstances. Who are they?

2. How contented are you with your social circle at the moment?

| Very contented | Contented | Neutral | Discontented | Very discontented |
|---|---|---|---|---|
| 1 | 2 | 3 | 4 | 5 |

3. What are the most important qualities you look for in a friend? Circle five (or more) descriptors from the list below.

| | | |
|---|---|---|
| Loyal | Unique | Authentic |
| Caring | Thoughtful | Encouraging |
| Funny | Entertaining | Affectionate |
| Reliable | Relatable | Easygoing |
| Empathetic | Comforting | Considerate |

**4.** Think about your current friendships. How well do the words you've identified above align with the people in your life right now?

| **Write each trait here** | **Score out of 10** – how well is this represented in your current friendships? |
|---|---|
| | |
| | |
| | |
| | |
| | |
| | |

COLOURING PAGE ➳

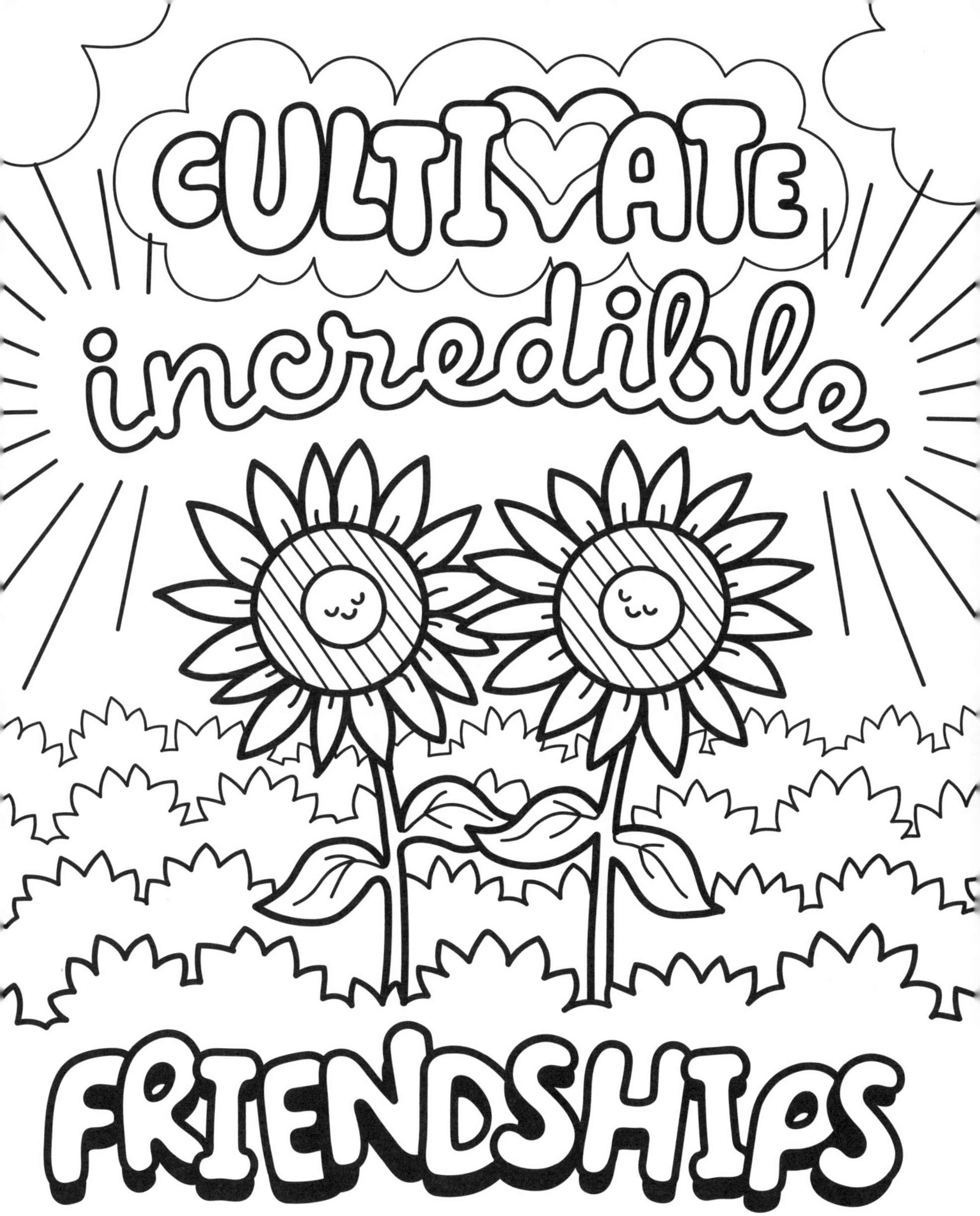
CULTIVATE
incredible
FRIENDSHIPS

## MEDIUM BATTERY QUESTIONS

**1.** What are your favourite ways to socialise? Write or draw them below.

**2.** How 'chronic illness-friendly' are the social activities you identified above? How might you adjust them to make them more accessible?

**3.** Which of the following access needs would benefit you in social settings? Highlight your answers from the choices below.

Quiet environment

Socialising from home

Outdoors

Indoors

Wearing a face mask and/ or social distancing

Wheelchair accessible

Plenty of seating

Allergen-friendly food

One-to-one catch-ups

Group gatherings

Activity-based with less talking (e.g. watching a movie)

Solo activities but done together (e.g. reading)

More talking, less activity

Set start and end time to aid pacing

Flexible end time depending on how you're feeling

Quiet room/somewhere to lie down

Somewhere linked with a special interest

Add your own here:

..........................................................

4. Are your friends aware of your access needs? If not, how might you describe them when you're making plans?

**My access needs are...**

5. This or that? When you're not physically with your friends, what are your preferred communication styles? Circle the ones that appeal to you.

| | | |
|---|---|---|
| **Catching up little and often** | or | **bigger, less frequent catch-ups?** |
| **Talking on the phone** | or | **messaging?** |
| **Digital communication** | or | **screen-free (e.g. letters/ postcards) communication?** |
| **Deep chats** | or | **light-hearted distraction?** |
| **Full-focus conversations** | or | **multitasking (e.g. chatting while eating lunch)?** |

**6.** What do you truly want out of a friendship? Rank the below factors in order, with 1 representing the most important and 5 representing the least important things to you.

- Somebody to enjoy fun activities with
- Emotional support and connection
- A person you can relate to
- Somebody who can make you laugh and entertain you
- Affection and closeness

**7.** Having time to ourselves is just as important as socialising, especially for introverts or ambiverts who need to recharge their social battery as well as their physical battery. In an ideal world, how much of your time would you spend with others and how much by yourself? Draw and label this split on this pie-chart (e.g. 75% alone, 25% with others, 50/50 split, or anything in between).

**8.** Do any of your friends also have a chronic illness or energy-limiting condition, and/or do you want to meet new people who you can relate to?

**9.** Are you part of the online chronic illness community? If so, note down your favourite content creators, hashtags, or virtual groups here.

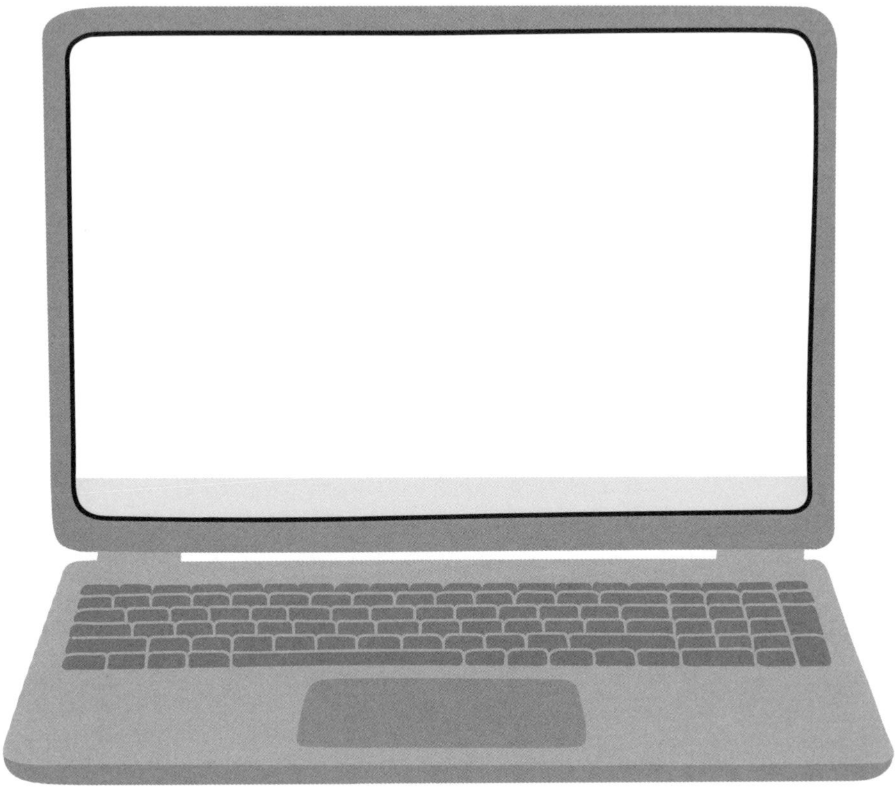

**10.** Our conditions can sometimes make us forget or doubt how much value we can bring to a friendship. Annotate this drawing to look like you, and label it with all the qualities that make you a great friend to others. Aim for a minimum of five – there will be more than you may think.

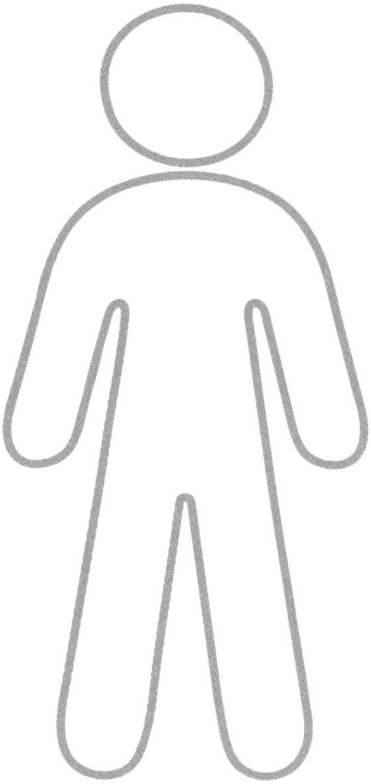

# 'BETTER' BATTERY QUESTIONS

1. Let's think about your boundaries. Sometimes we're willing to let things slide with our good friends to try and keep the peace, but tricky or problematic friendships can drain our limited energy. Let's think about which of the following hypothetical situations would be a deal-breaker, and how you would respond to them.

| **Tricky situation** | **Is this a deal-breaker for you?** | **How will you respond?** |
|---|---|---|
| Plans are made that aren't suitable for your access needs | | |
| A friend offers unsolicited advice | | |
| There are feelings of awkwardness or discomfort when you talk about your condition | | |
| A friend expresses regret or longing for things the way they were before you acquired your condition | | |
| Plans you've paced or prepared for are cancelled by them at the last minute | | |

Guidance on handling and responding to tricky scenarios like these can be found in Chapters 4 and 5 of my book *How to Do Life with a Chronic Illness*.

2. How comfortable or uncomfortable do you feel about having difficult conversations or raising concerns with your friends? If there is discomfort here, where do you think it's coming from?

3. When you have an energy-limiting condition, spending time with others takes planning and pacing. Examples might include packing a bag the day before with any necessary medical supplies, allowing rest breaks while getting ready, and clearing your diary the following day(s) while you recover. What adjustments would make socialising more accessible for you?

**4.** Word search. Find the following words below – are there any that jump out at you before the others?

| C | B | Q | G | C | I | M | G | K | Q | S | Q | K | U | K |
|---|---|---|---|---|---|---|---|---|---|---|---|---|---|---|
| K | O | F | B | I | I | V | V | L | S | O | A | Z | N | R |
| S | G | N | T | O | H | K | M | P | W | C | A | T | O | F |
| V | Q | Z | N | N | N | Y | C | P | H | I | R | U | I | W |
| B | D | J | C | E | E | Z | Y | U | K | A | D | I | T | R |
| Y | C | E | S | S | C | M | G | F | E | L | O | O | A | R |
| B | C | B | Z | P | L | T | Y | F | R | I | E | N | D | S |
| T | R | O | P | P | U | S | I | O | K | S | M | D | I | M |
| N | L | V | B | S | F | Y | Z | O | J | I | D | S | L | D |
| H | B | O | Z | U | J | T | A | W | N | N | G | G | A | J |
| Q | R | Y | N | U | B | V | Q | F | C | G | E | H | V | E |
| S | X | U | W | B | C | Y | M | V | A | D | E | Q | Q | E |
| N | U | B | I | G | L | H | U | W | R | V | C | I | I | A |
| F | V | W | I | D | O | X | T | S | Y | M | A | S | R | B |
| Q | U | P | U | L | G | F | U | I | G | N | Z | K | J | K |

Friends Socialising Support Validation

Connection Fun Enjoyment

**5.** **Journal prompt:** What does your social circle look like, and what do you want it to be?

- How have your friendships and social life changed since acquiring your condition?
- Have there been any situations where your friends have let you down, or others where they have really shown up for you?

- Are there any needs you feel are being unmet in your current friendships, and how do you see your social circle evolving in the future?

# SECTION 6
# THOUGHTS FOR THE FUTURE

THINKING about the future can feel a little overwhelming sometimes. During the years following my diagnosis, I genuinely thought my life was over. I wouldn't allow myself to think about the future, because with such an unpredictable illness trajectory, I truly thought that all my best days were behind me. But I was so wrong. This time in my life was simply the beginning of a new chapter. My twenties have looked vastly different to how I once imagined them for myself, but they have been interwoven with so much laughter and fulfilment, even alongside the struggles.

In my early years of chronic illness, people would often try to make me feel better by telling me I could still do *anything* I put my mind to, even when clearly that was far from the case. Instead of motivating me and lighting a fire in my belly, as they were intended to, hearing these things led me to feel insecure about how my situation was being perceived by others. I wish there had been somebody to tell me that who I was, and how I was doing things at that moment, was more than good enough. I wish I had known that even with such limited energy, there was still so much time and opportunity ahead of me.

Despite this, it's important to recognise that not all of us are on an even playing field here. We don't all have the same level of autonomy over how we spend our time and energy and the plans we make for the future. You may have a very severe form of your condition or live with a degenerative or terminal illness. You may have parenting or caregiving responsibilities and have to take care of others' needs as well as your own. You may be living in financial uncertainty or falling between the gaps in social support. We all have our privileges, and we all have our burdens. Often, we see only a fraction of the story on social media, or even when we meet people in person. It's so important that we treat each other with kindness and empathy, even when our trajectories seem very different from each other. Our wants and expectations for the future are as unique as we each are ourselves.

Therefore, I'm not here to tell you that you're capable of absolutely anything, and that hard work and a can-do attitude will overcome the very real barriers you face. Like with many other elements we've explored throughout this journal, it serves us best to focus on doing what we can with what we have. However, in my experience, living with a chronic illness and having only a limited number of usable minutes or hours per day does have one unique bonus – it highlights the things that truly matter to us, and the things in life that feel *worth* exchanging our valuable energy for. For me, and perhaps for you, it's led me to consider what I truly want my future to look like, rather than what society had made me think I *should* want my future to look like.

In this section, we're going to gently explore what you may want out of the future too...but not in terms of your physical capabilities. Of course, many of us would (metaphorically) jump at the chance to improve our energy levels or reduce our symptoms, and I truly hope that happens for you, but the uncertainty of many conditions means we can't necessarily bank on these things happening. So instead, let's broaden the lens we're looking through. Let's identify our personal hopes and preferences for how we want to spend our energy and what we want to strive for, while accommodating our access needs and honouring any other commitments or barriers we're contending with.

If you are newly diagnosed or have recently experienced some setbacks in your health, this section may feel a little too tricky to engage with at the moment. If that's the case, I suggest you put this to one side for now and come back to it later. And regardless of who you are or the circumstances you find yourself in, may I offer you a gentle reminder? I hope you always remember that where you are and what you're doing now is more than good enough. Your output does not define your worth, and you're never obligated to make radical changes to your way of life. You don't have to mould your behaviour to meet the expectations of those around you, or the world at large. Instead, let's focus on identifying the things that truly matter to you and might bring you joy in the future, and figure out some accessible steps to help us get there.

# LOW BATTERY QUESTIONS

**1.** At present, how often do you think about the future?

| **0%** | **100%** |
|---|---|
| Not at all | All the time |

**2.** When you think about the future, how does it make you feel? Mark or colour in the emotions below.

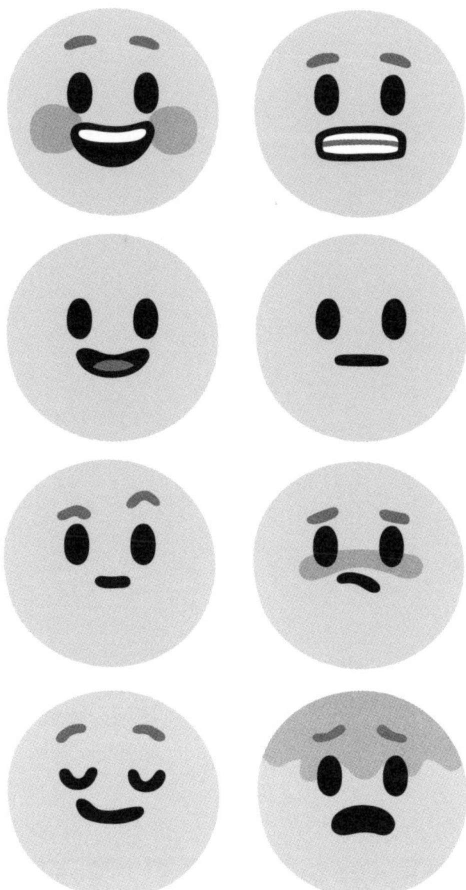

Excited | Apprehensive
Optimistic | Neutral
Intrigued | Uncertain
Empowered | Fearful

**3.** This or that? Circle the words that most describe the future you would like for yourself (or mark the space somewhere in between).

| | | |
|---|---|---|
| **Calm** | or | **stimulating?** |
| **Stable** | or | **variable?** |
| **Minimalist** | or | **maximalist?** |
| **Routine** | or | **unpredictable?** |
| **Slow living** | or | **faster paced?** |

**4.** If you had to choose just one of your personality traits to carry into the future, which one would it be?

COLOURING PAGE »→

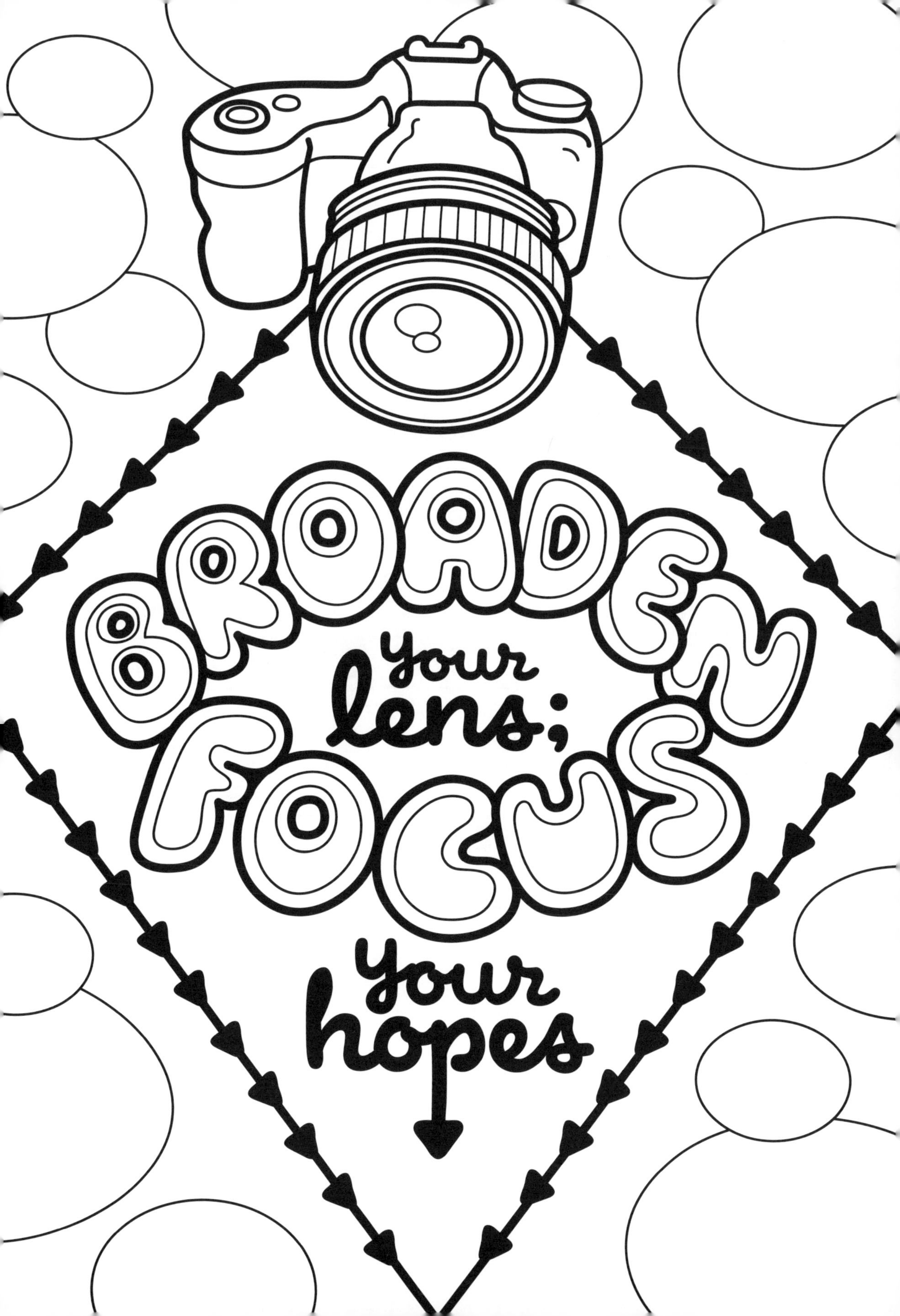
BROADEN your lens;
FOCUS your hopes

## MEDIUM BATTERY QUESTIONS

**1.** If you had to write a newspaper headline for your chronic illness journey so far, what would it be?

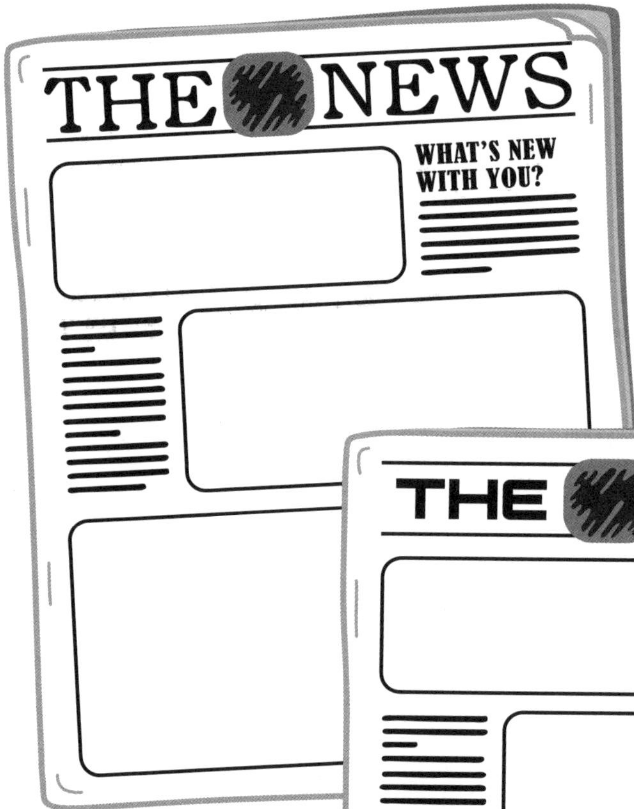


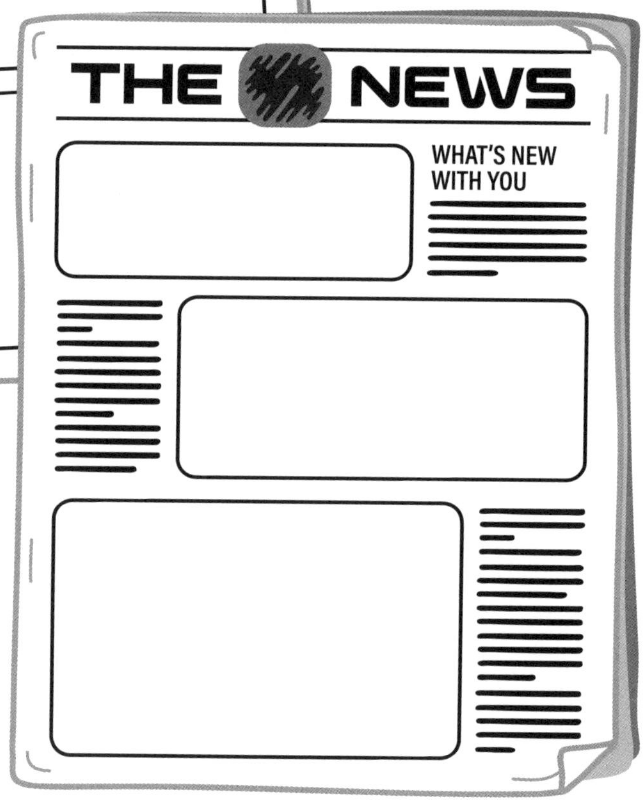


**2.** If you can, think about yourself in 20 years' time. What would you like the newspaper headline to read then?

**3.** At this moment in time, what are your goals for the future? Remember, we're not necessarily thinking about health-related or physical factors here, but the things that you as an individual would like for yourself.

1

2

3

**4.** What made you choose these goals? For each of them, take a moment to reflect on why you want to reach them and what this may tell you about yourself.

1

2

3

**5.** Now, let's think about any goals for the immediate future. Is there anything you can adjust in the here and now that would improve your quality of life?

Examples could include adding more rest breaks into your day, drinking more water, making space for a hobby you enjoy, scheduling a regular time to speak with your friends...

**6.** An implementation intention is a plan you make ahead of time, to describe how you will implement a certain habit. According to the Atomic Habits theory, the following sentence offers a framework for getting specific about how you will introduce a behaviour into your life:

I will [BEHAVIOUR] at [TIME] in [LOCATION]

For example, I will drink a glass of water at the beginning of my day in the kitchen. Thinking about the goal you have chosen, complete your own sentence here...

I will .................................... at .................... in ........................................

**7.** If your condition makes it difficult to plan for the future or anticipate how you will be feeling, you may find habit stacking more appealing instead. Habit stacking is when we link our new behaviours with routine behaviours we perform every day, rather than putting specific time aside. Linking them with our everyday routines, such as brushing our teeth or putting the kettle on, can help them become a habit. This sentence provides a framework:

After [CURRENT HABIT], I will [NEW HABIT]

For example, after I get dressed, I will lie down and rest for ten minutes. With your goal in mind, complete your own sentence here...

After ........................................ I will ..................................................

Questions 6 and 7 have been informed by *Atomic Habits* by James Clear. The book is definitely written for the non-disabled gaze, but contains some excellent advice and further reading if you're interested in the science of habits!

**8.** Are there any ways you could customise your environment to make it easier or more enjoyable to take steps towards your goals? Draw your answer here.

**9.** Are there any ways the people around you could make it easier or more enjoyable to take steps towards your goals? How might you communicate that to them?

**10.** How will you weave rest and pacing into your steps towards your goals? Write down three adaptations/adjustments below.

1

2

3

# 'BETTER' BATTERY QUESTIONS

**1.** We are worth so much more than our output and accomplishments, but in our achievement-driven world it can be so easy to forget this. At the moment, how much of your self-worth comes from your output or accomplishments?

**0 1 2 3 4 5 6 7 8 9 10**

None of my self-worth — All of my self-worth

**2.** Consider your answer above. Why do you think you've selected the number you have? Is there anything in your environment or upbringing that might have hooked or unhooked you from the belief that your productivity defines your worth?

**3.** Now think about if a chronically ill friend had said to you what you've just written above. What advice would you give them?

**4.** As we all know, but can be prone to forget, life isn't about making tangible accomplishments or keeping up with others. If you struggle to adopt a new habit or don't manage to achieve one of your goals in the future, how will you show kindness to yourself? Draw or illustrate your answer here.

**5.** On a similar note, it can be immensely satisfying to live in the present and appreciate where we are right now. How will you enjoy and celebrate your everyday wins in life? Draw or illustrate your answer here.

**6.** **Journal prompt:** What do you want out of the future?

- How do you feel about the future right now? What matters most to you in life, and has this changed since you became ill?
- How will you think about your future with compassion, while keeping grounded in the here and now?
- What could you do to make your goals more achievable while taking good care of yourself and managing your condition?

(more space overleaf!)

# TIME CAPSULE 3

Use this space to record information about you, your chronic illness, and your health and wellbeing at this moment in time.

**What is the date and time?**

**How is your physical health today?**

**How is your mental health today?**

**What are three things you feel grateful for today?**

**What challenges are you facing at the moment?**

**Time to thought-dump. What's on your mind today?**

# A LETTER TO YOUR FUTURE SELF

If you read my book *How to Do Life with a Chronic Illness*, you may know that I write letters to my future self. Sitting down to capture your thoughts and feelings in that very moment is such a powerful way to self-reflect, and also gives your future self the gift of opening your letters from the past and experiencing your words in a whole new light. It's also an incredible way of documenting life experiences that you want future you to hold on to, before the pesky brain fog has a chance to get to them.

Therefore, your final activity is to write a letter to your future self, even if you just try it this one time. Use the questions below to help you get started, then grab some paper and an envelope. Write down your message (as long or short as you like), seal up the envelope and write the date you'll open it on the front, and put it away until the time comes. Try, really try, not to peek at it before the date you've decided on comes around. Trust me, it'll feel worth it.

**1.** I'm writing a letter for my future self to open in...

6 months 1 year 2 years 5 years 10 years

**2.** Therefore, the date I will open my letter will be...

**3.** Use these prompts to make notes or drafts before you begin writing your letter.

**What does life look like for you at the moment?**

**What brings you joy?**

**What struggles are you facing?**

**What are you most proud of right now?**

**What do you wish you knew about your future self?**

**What do you want your future self to remember about this point in your life?**

Happy writing!

# FINAL REFLECTIONS

AT the beginning of this journal, I spoke about how little control we seem to have over our conditions, and how difficult this can be to deal with. However, I hope that by spending time within these pages, you've been able to reconnect with you – the real, three-dimensional person who is doing their best to live the life they choose alongside managing their chronic illness. No matter how small they may seem, there are always choices we can make, and ways of making our lives feel a little more like our own. We can't choose our disease trajectory, symptoms, or prognosis, but through the tiniest decisions, we really do have some autonomy over how we show up and express ourselves, and how we Do Life alongside our conditions.

More than anything, I want to say thank you for spending your valuable time and energy with me as you've worked your way through this journal. I hope you've learned something new about yourself while enjoying these activities, or reconnected with a part of yourself that you thought had been lost. If not, I just hope you've enjoyed spending some time looking inwardly and focusing on self-reflection – something that we often don't get to spend as much time doing as we should, but can be immensely gratifying.

Before you turn the page and skim through the further resources I've provided, I hope you'll take a moment right now to feel proud of yourself. It's not easy to live with a chronic illness, especially in a world that frequently makes us feel as though we're lesser than non-disabled people. But if you ask me, making your way through life at your own pace and being your brilliant, beautiful self is one of the greatest acts of rebellion of them all. I'm proud of you, because you're you. I hope you're proud of being you, too.

# USEFUL RESOURCES

## Helplines and support

If you're seeking support for your mental wellbeing but need this to come from somebody who understands the physical challenges you're facing, the following organisations may be able to help:

**Pain Concern Helpline**
help@painconcern.org.uk
0300 123 0789

**CISFA (Chronic Illness Support For All) UK**
www.cisfauk.org

**ME Connect Helpline (The ME Association)**
meconnect@meassociation.org.uk
0344 5765326

**SHOUT**
https://giveusashout.org
Text 85258

**Scope Helpline**
helpline@scope.org.uk
0808 800 3333

## Social media communities

There's an incredible online chronic illness community out there, full of people who I truly believe are making the world a better place. Here are examples of some hashtags for you to find and connect with others who have similar lived experiences to you:

- #ChronicIllness
- #ChronicPain
- #Spoonie
- #DisabledBloggers
- #NEISVoid [No End In Sight Void]
- #InvisibleIllness
- #ButYouDontLookSick
- #DisabledAndCute
- #BabeWithAMobilityAid

You can also...

- Use the name of your condition and research any specific hashtags – for example, #MECFS and #PWME [People With ME] for those with ME/CFS.
- Include your hobbies or interests to find online communities – for example, #DisabledWriter, #ChronicallyIllCreatives, #DisabledFashion, #AccessibleTheatre.
- Start your own movement! If you enjoy content creation and can't quite find what you're looking for, decide on a username and hashtag and start building your happy place. There may well be other lovely people looking for the same thing...

## Further reading

- *Pace Yourself* by Amy Arthur
- *Atomic Habits* by James Clear
- *Daring Greatly* by Brené Brown

- *Crippled* by Frances Ryan
- *Sacred Rest* by Saundra Dalton-Smith
- *All Tangled Up in Autism and Chronic Illness* by Charli Clement
- *University and Chronic Illness: A Survival Guide* by Pippa Stacey
- *Occupational Therapy, Disability Activism, and Me* by Georgia Vine

## How to Do Life with a Chronic Illness

Reclaim Your Identity, Create Independence, and Find Your Way Forward

**Pippa Stacey**

*'I know that living with a chronic illness in this inaccessible world is tough. Trust me, I know. But you deserve to find peace and contentment just as much as anybody else. So welcome to your one-stop guide on how to make the most of life alongside your condition, in a way that truly works for you.'*

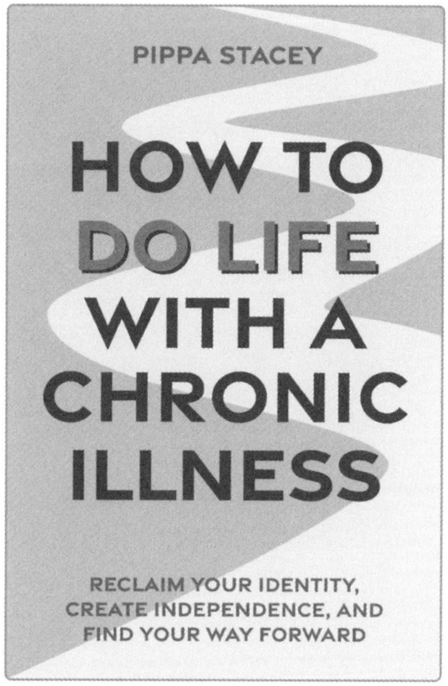


Chronic illness affects everybody differently, but we all share the goal of living meaningfully and making the most of what we have. This book exists to help you take accessible steps towards that goal and build a life that truly feels like yours.

Instead of focusing on the medical side of long-term conditions, this book dives into the important parts of everyday living that often go unspoken about, from practical advice on friendships, dating and independent living, to more reflective guidance on rediscovering your identity and learning to self-advocate.

Between these pages, you'll find bespoke information and resources curated through 10+ years of lived experience, alongside words of wisdom from diverse contributors and subject experts. This book also contains journal prompts, resource lists, and (perhaps most importantly) words of comfort and validation that people with life-altering conditions simply do not hear enough.

ISBN 978 1 80501 017 3 | eISBN 978 1 80501 018 0 | AUDIOBOOK ISBN 978 1 39981 633 5